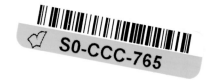

Basic
Herbs
and
Simple Remedies

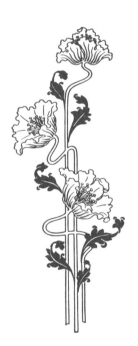

by Janet Vickers

1

Basic Herbs and Simple Remedies
by
Janet Vickers

Eighth Printing — **October 1992**

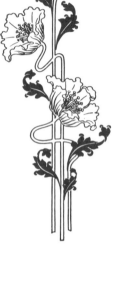

Copyright © **1980 by Janet Vickers**
all rights reserved

Published by: **NuYu Publishing**
a division of NuYu Enterprises
Box 8432, Station F
Calgary, Alberta, Canada T2J 2V5

Canadian Cataloguing in Publication Data

Vickers, Janet
Basic herbs and simple remedies

Rev. ed. —

1st ed. 1980 published under title: Let's talk basic herbs and simple remedies.
ISBN: 0-919845-88-6

1. Herbs — Therapeutic use. 2. Materia medica, Vegetable. 3. Herbal cosmetics. I. Title. II. Title: Let's talk basic herbs and simple remedies.

RS164.V53 1990   615/.321   C90-097168-1

Photography by
Patricia Holdsworth
Patricia Holdsworth Photography
Regina, Saskatchewan

Designed, Printed and Produced in Canada by:
Centax Books, a Division of PrintWest Communications
Publishing Director and Photo Designer:
  Margo Embury
1150 Eighth Avenue, Regina, Saskatchewan
  Canada S4R 1C9
(306) 525-2304   FAX (306) 757-2439

CONTENTS

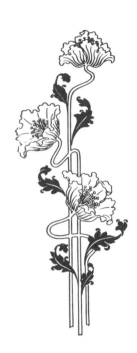

3

ACKNOWLEDGEMENTS

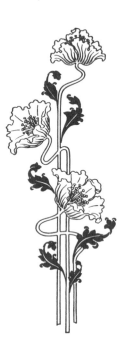

There are always people who make the writing of a book easier, their support, enthusiasm, encouragement and help in so many ways add up to the finished effort. My sincere thanks to Marjorie Burakoff who typed the manuscript and gave helpful suggestions. To the many friends who gave me their simple remedies for use in the book. For the Heritage that is ours and the abundance of the Earth in providing us with all that we need. For my husband Hugh, who suggested the book for the help it could be to everyone, especially families. Finally, to our two sons, Michael and Austin, without whom throughout the years we wouldn't have had anyone to try out the Basic Herbs and Simple Remedies.

Janet Vickers

ABOUT HERBS AND THIS BOOK

For thousands of years man and animals have relied on the plant kingdom for food, shelter and medicine. As we study history we find many references to medicinal plants that are still being used today. There is a revival of interest at the present time in plant medicines, as people from all age groups realize that the remedies grandma used really worked. Plant remedies have passed the test of time. The ancient Greeks, Romans, Chinese and Native Indians all have a history of the effectiveness of herbs in the maintenance of health.

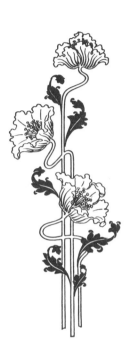

The early settlers to the Americas used old herbal remedies brought with them that had been handed down through several generations. They also learned of many new ones from the North American Indians.

There are thousands of herbs on the land and in the ocean, put there for the use of man. This book contains information on just a few of them. During my lectures across Canada and the United States many people asked for a simple book with easy-to-follow directions. I decided to gather up the remedies that were given to me over the years (tried and tested on my own family and friends) and put together this simple book. Since many of these have been handed down, I'm sure you will recognize some of them.

The first part of the book you will find devoted to some basic herbs that have multiple actions, are nutritive and have earned the respect of early generations, many times through trial and error. Already dependent upon the plant world for food and shelter, how natural it was for early man to also rely on it for medicine.

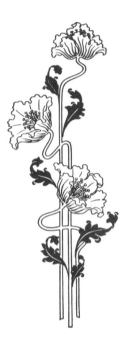

The rest of the book is divided into simple remedies utilizing everyday herbs, vegetables and fruits for both external and internal use. You will find information on vitamins and minerals and which foods contain them. There are also beauty aids utilizing nature's gifts and healthful substitutes for refined and processed foods.

There are many fine books written on herbs and nutrition to be found in your local health food stores, far more detailed and technical than this one. For those of you interested in studying herbs in greater depth there are now courses available through educational institutions across the country.

Many people, over the years, helped me raise my children in a natural way by sharing their knowledge with me. One dear lady of 94 who was a pioneer in Canada's North, used to spend hours telling me of all the natural remedies she learned from living and working with the Indian people. She looked so healthy, happy and contented, had a firm stride and obviously enjoyed life. I asked her questions on health and attitude. She said the following — "I eat mostly the bounties

6

of Nature, grow my own vegetables, bake my own whole-grain bread, exercise in the fresh air, breathe deeply to keep relaxed, think good, positive thoughts (especially of others), help anyone I can, have faith in God (give thanks everyday for my blessings) and keep well with herbs and other simple remedies. You see," she said, "It's really easy, just keep your life simple." Dear readers, her sentiments are also mine. Life can be simple and simply beautiful. To Florence Hansen and all the kind people who shared with me, I dedicate this simple, little book. It was not intended to replace medical attention when needed, but rather to let you know that there are simple kitchen herbs that can help you, both inside and out.

Janet Vickers

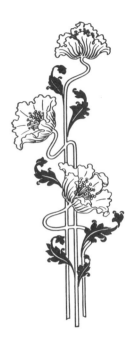

ALFALFA
Medicago sativa

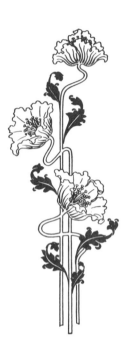

This herb was believed named by the Arabs. It means father of all foods. It was used in Greece 500 years B.C. The United States alone produces millions of tons each year. The roots of Alfalfa extend down into the earth extracting valuable vitamins and minerals from the soil. Chlorophyll is one of the main ingredients of Alfalfa. It also provides a source of potassium, magnesium, phosphorus, calcium, plus vitamin A, vitamin C, vitamin K, vitamin D and vitamin E. It greatly improves poor appetite and is a light diuretic and general tonic. Nursing mothers could benefit greatly from drinking 2 or 3 cups daily because of the protein content. Use 1 tsp. per cup, add boiling water and allow to steep 5 minutes, strain and drink.

When Alfalfa is sprouted, it becomes an excellent source of greens containing valuable amino acids and is especially valuable during the winter months to replace lettuce in salads. Incidentally, sprouts are really more nutritious than lettuce at any time of year because of their high protein and iron content. To prepare sprouts, take a 2-quart mason jar and put 3 tbsp. of Alfalfa seeds inside. Cover the opening with either a screen (mesh) or cheesecloth. Cover seeds with water and leave overnight. The next day drain through the cover, rinse seeds once or twice (using warm water), put one of hubby's socks (washed) on the jar to keep it dark, then turn the jar on its side. Rinse

8

twice daily until the sprouts are desired length. Second day take off sock and put the jar in sunlight if possible. This brings out the chlorophyll and turns them green. Used for sandwiches, they are delicious, nutritious and economical.

ALOE
Aloe vera

This graceful plant is very decorative in the home as well as being easy to raise. Its uses as a healing plant are unending. Basically there are 200 varieties of Aloe. The species I'm referring to now is the Aloe Vera, a member of the Lily family. It looks rather like a cactus. It actually is a hardy plant but dislikes the coldest parts of the house. People in Texas and Arizona use the jelly-like substance from the leaves to massage into their hair and into their skin. It acts like a conditioner for the scalp and as a remedy for sunburn it is indispensable. Skin infections of all kinds benefit from Aloe — burns, stings, poison ivy, eczema, athlete's foot. To use externally, peel leaves back, remove yellow sticky substance directly under leaf. Apply clear gel to affected area.

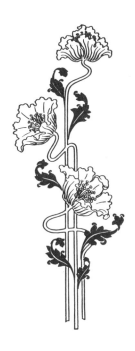

9

ANISE
Pimpinella anisum

This valuable and versatile herb is
believed to have originated in the Middle
East. The oil of Anise has an aromatic
odor and gives much flavor when added to
baked goods. It is often used for the
making of confectionery. Its medicinal use
is varied, it helps prevent gas in the
stomach and bowels, is excellent for
nausea and if used in steam to help
control an excessively oily skin, has no
competitor. The seeds and fruit are used
for this. Make an infusion (tea) by
steeping 1 dessert spoon of cut or crushed
herb to 1 cup of boiling water; allow to
cool, strain before drinking.

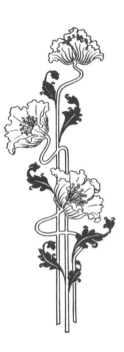

AVENS ROOT
Geum urbenum

Also referred to as Chocolate root, this
herb was highly regarded by early English
herbalists for its antiseptic qualities and
use as a general restorative and tonic. It
was also recommended as a gargle for sore
throat. In folk medicine it was given for
the improvement of the complexion as
well as a correction for the digestive
system. To make an infusion (tea) 1 oz.
powdered herb to 16 oz. boiling water is
used and taken by the ounce three times
daily after meals.

BLACK COHOSH
Cimicifuga racemosa

Useful for female complaints, especially
during menopause. It helps to bring on
menstrual flow and helps flushing. It
brings about balance in the circulation and
is beneficial for high blood pressure. Use
as an infusion twice daily.

BLESSED THISTLE
Cnicus benedictus

Early herbalists regarded and revered
Blessed Thistle as a remedy for smallpox.
The name blessed indicates it was
considered special. Its later uses included
both internal and external applications.
Folk medicine refers to this plant as a
cure-all. It was used to treat headaches,
fevers, infections internally and applied to
skin eruptions externally.

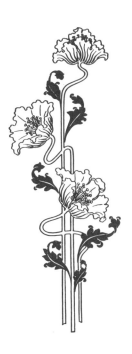

BLUE VIOLET LEAVES
Viola odorata

Early English herbalists and pharmacists
alike used the violet for the making of a
syrup which was used in the treatment of
consumption. It can still be found today as
an ingredient in cough drops or cough
syrup. Ancients also found value in the
violet as a treatment for skin problems,
this would account for its inclusion in
cosmetic formulas and ointments for the
purpose of treating boils, psoriasis and
excema. An infusion of 1 oz. violet leaves
to 16 oz. boiling water can be made and
used as a gargle for a sore throat as well
as a soothing drink to relieve headaches.

BORAGE
Borago officinalis

Found extensively in England, both flowers and leaves are used to make a simple tea which, in turn, can be used internally as a blood cleanser, for coughs to release phlegm and as a gargle for a sore throat. For external use, apply tea with small sponge to sores and skin abrasions, insect bites, rashes, etc.

BURDOCK
Arctium lappa

Roots, leaves and seeds can be used for a wide variety of disorders, both internal and external. Found in ditches and on roadsides, Burdock is believed to have its origin in Europe. Burdock is excellent for purifying the blood, aiding in conditions such as acne, eczema, boils and rashes. It also helps the flow of urine. Take as a simple tea several times daily for any skin problems. Externally, Burdock can be made into a salve and applied to wounds, burns, swellings and hemorrhoids.

CATNIP
Nepeta cataria

Catnip is very useful for pain due to gas, spasms, griping and colic in children. A very soothing drink can be made by steeping Catnip (1 tsp. per cup) and adding a tiny touch of honey; this helps to promote sleep.

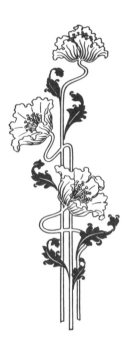

CAYENNE
Capsicum minimum

Herbalists everywhere sing praises for this valuable herb. Most households have it and use it in hot dishes such as chili. Apart from its culinary magic, it is excellent as a medicine. This herb usually is cultivated in tropical regions, Africa, South America, West Indies. There are also several species available. The best medicinal properties occur in African Bird Pepper. Your local herb shop should have this. Poor circulation, congestion, chills, feeling of low energy and sore throats due to colds are all benefited by the use of Cayenne. Even though it feels hot, it is not to be confused with Black Pepper. In its function, Cayenne is soothing and particularly loved by the natives in the countries it is grown in. This herb, to them, is like Ginseng to the Oriental, a panacea, (good for everything).

CELERY
Apium graveolens

When you are feeling upset and overtired or nervous, reach for the celery. Long used as a nerve tonic, it is also excellent to nibble on during extremely hot weather. It keeps the blood cool and contains organic sodium which in turn works with calcium to prevent blood thickening. Celery also contains natural iron that does not create constipation like its synthetic counterpart. Dieters may appreciate it because it helps to satisfy hunger pains. If celery is put through a juicer and blended with carrot juice, ¾ carrot to ¼ celery it makes a delightful and nutritious drink.

13

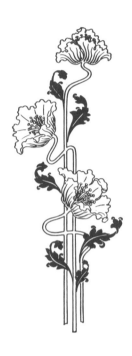

CHAMOMILE
Anthemis nobile

Found extensively in Europe, this plant has been used for centuries for nervous complaints and as a mild tonic. It helps to increase appetite, relieves flatulence and is especially beneficial for colicky babies. Make an infusion of the flowers and allow to steep. Take 1 or 2 cups daily, 1 cup before bedtime to promote sleep. If given for babies, 3 or 4 tsp. daily is sufficient.

CHAPARRAL
Larrea tridentata

Found in the desert regions of the United States Chaparral has a strong bitter taste and odor. Used traditionally by Indians to cleanse and purge the body internally and as a wash externally for the healing of sores. It is presently the subject of study in various Universities for the purpose of identifying potential medicinal ingredients. Some Navajo Indians in Arizona today, still regard Chaparral as a cure-all especially in the treatment of skin problems. Chaparral is available in leaves or capsule form. If taken as a tea a little honey will help to alleviate the bitter taste.

COMFREY
Symphytum officinale

Considered by many to be one of the most useful plants in existence. It is believed to have had its origin in southern Russia. Another name for it is Knitbone due to its amazing ability to hasten the mending of broken bones. Veterinarians in the past used it to treat external wounds, sores, abrasions and gave it as fodder because the leaves contain a good source of protein as well as vitamins and minerals. Early herbalists and the medical profession used it for the treatment of pulmonary conditions, asthma, bronchitis and intestinal upset.

Modern day practitioners use it externally for insect bites, ulcers and burns. The leaves contain little juice, but a thick mucous-like substance. Comfrey is easy to grow and both leaves and roots can be used. If roots are used, make a decoction of 1 oz. crushed root to 1 quart of water (Cold water poured over root, bring to boil, let simmer 20 minutes, cool and strain.) If dried leaves are used, 1 pint of boiling water to 1 oz. of leaves. Scientists are studying the effect of Comfrey over long term internal use.

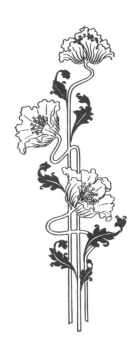

CULVERS ROOT
Veronicastrum virginicum

The American Indians are credited with discovering the therapeutic properties of Culvers Root. It was included in tribal ceremonies and was considered a blood cleanser by the Chippewas.

Early herbalists believed it to be valuable in the treatment of liver dysfunction and also used it to rectify digestive disorders. Modern day practitioners use it for the same purposes. It is available from herb shops and is taken as a tea.

DANDELION
Taraxacum officinale

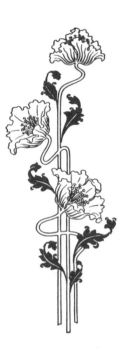

Most people curse the plant because it has an affinity for front lawns. It originally was considered a European import but it makes an appearance in all temperate climates. On the Continent the leaves are added to salads and are an excellent source of Vitamins A and C. The root is used in the making of a cereal beverage and has a coffee-like flavor. This beverage was in fact used in Europe during World War II as a coffee substitute. Medicinally, Dandelion is used by herbalists as a mild laxative and overall tonic especially good for the liver and gallbladder. Early herbalists also used it as a treatment for billious attacks, neuralgia, skin eruptions, gout and water retention. An infusion can be made by adding 1 oz. dried flowers to 16 oz. water. Two or three cups taken daily is said to be good for digestion. Caution: Be sure not to use Dandelions sprayed with chemicals.

FENUGREEK
Trigonella foenum-graecum

Sprouted as seeds, Fenugreek is delightful in salads. The seeds made into a tea are excellent for sinus problems and effective in relieving flatulence and upset stomach due to overeating. In the springtime anyone suffering from allergies would benefit greatly by drinking Fenugreek tea 3 times daily. The seeds made into a poultice are excellent for drawing out infections of the skin.

16

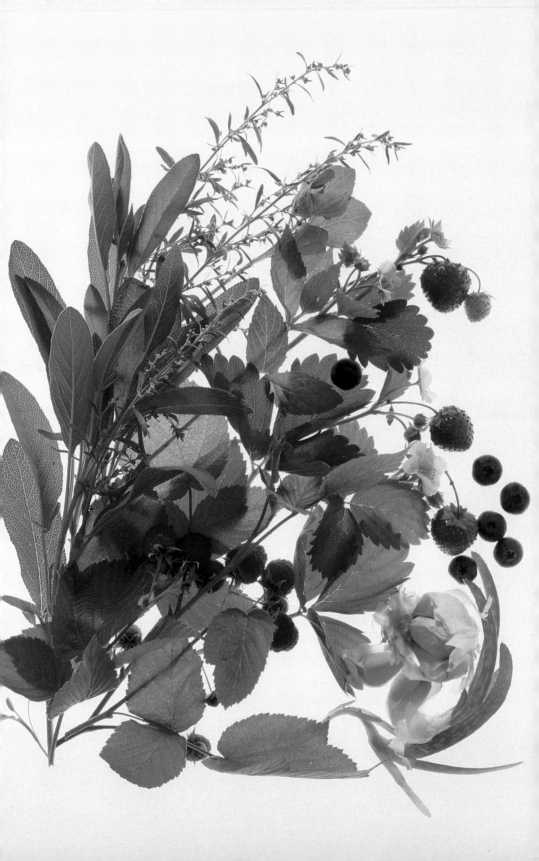

SIMPLE REMEDIES
Raspberry Leaves, Raspberries
Blueberries
Strawberries
Garlic
Aloe Vera
Horehound
Mint
Sage

GARLIC
Allium sativum

Most of you are familiar with garlic as a
flavoring agent on roasts, etc. It is much
maligned because of its so called offensive
odor, but if I had the choice of one herb in
the kitchen, it would be this one. Garlic is
a member of the lily family. It is
extremely high in sulphur and has an
active ingredient called Allicin. Used by
the ancient Egyptians, Chinese, Greeks
and Romans, there is no doubt of its
medicinal value. During the black plague
it was reported in England, one household
escaped the dreaded disease because of
Garlic being used by the family. It is
considered an antibiotic. In the Second
World War, British people were paid high
prices for Garlic by the government. It was
used for poultices for wounded soldiers, a
wonderful antiseptic. Today it is used as a
blood pressure normalizer and is also
effective in bronchial disorders, flatulence,
hardening of the arteries and as a general
strengthener of the body. If the Garlic
clove is slivered into just enough milk to
mix and then taken at night, the odor has
usually disappeared by morning.

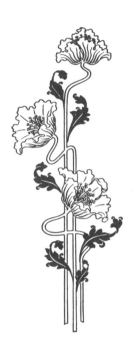

GINGER ROOT
Zingiber officinale

Widely cultivated in tropical climates.
Ginger has a variety of uses in both food
and medicine. Used as a flavoring agent, it
also contains some essential vitamins and
minerals as well as properties that
promote good digestion. Long considered a
valuable aid to motion sickness by

17

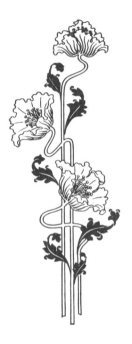

herbalists, it is now recognized by the scientific community as fact. Taken during menstruation, Ginger relieves cramping. It is also useful in warding off a cold as it brings warmth to the system. If Senna leaf tea is taken to relieve constipation, a pinch of ginger added to the tea prevents cramping. To relax nerves, take a small piece of Ginger root, grate it into 4 oz. of skim milk with 1 tsp. of sesame tahini.

GINSENG
Panax quinquefolius

Otherwise known as American Ginseng, it has earned the reputation of cure-all by Eastern and Western cultures alike. A different species than the Oriental Ginseng, it is still used by Orientals in the treatment of certain conditions. American Ginseng is a native of the United States and some parts of Canada. Russian and Chinese studies indicate it has the ability to eliminate radiation from the system and when used in combination with other herbs acts as a carrier and strengthens the body generally. There are many records of home remedies in which it is used for improved circulation, balancing of appetite and digestive problems. It is also said to promote mental vigor and alertness. The root of the Ginseng is slow growing and this contributes to the high cost. In Chinese herb shops the cost varies according to the age of the root.

GOLDEN SEAL
Hydrastis canadensis

It has been said of Golden Seal that it is worth its weight in gold and is aptly named. It is extremely useful for skin problems such as eczema, psoriasis, sores of any kind. To bathe affected parts, brew a tea of 1 tsp. to 16 oz. boiling water. Apply when cool as a wash. Excellent as a gargle for sore throats. For especially hard to heal sores (external), mix with equal parts of Myrrh. Make an ointment using a little vaseline as a base. Apply directly and cover with gauze.

HOPS
Humulus lupulus

Excellent as a mild sedative, warm tea can be taken 1 hour before retiring. Very relaxing for nervous stomach or tension headache. A mild tea can be made using 1 oz. Hops to 16 oz. boiling water. Allow to stand a few minutes, then strain. 1 cup before bedtime produces a good sleep with no harmful side effects.

HORSETAIL
Equisetum arvense

American Indians and early settlers used horsetail as a diuretic and to staunch excessive bleeding internally. English herbalists used it as an aid to kidney complaints and to reduce acidity of the stomach. Because of its high silicon content it helps to promote healthy hair, skin and nails. Externally it can be used to heal cuts and sores. To make a tea use 1 tsp. to 4 oz. of water.

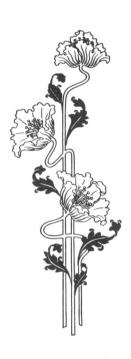

19

HYDRANGEA
Hydrangea arborescens

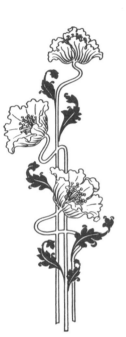

Hydrangea has been recognized for its ability to remove gravelly deposits and relieve the associated pain. The Cherokee Indians especially recognized its importance for the prevention of kidney stones. Both early and modern day herbalists used it as a general tonic and recommended it for the relief of rheumatism. Rutin, a substance valuable in improving capillary fragility is present in Hydrangea. A tea made of 1 oz. root to 16 oz. hot water and taken 2 oz. twice daily is recommended as a tonic. Honey can be added if desired.

HYSSOP
Hyssopus officinalis

An old Bible remedy and one used by the Romans as medicine and food. A member of the mint family, it contains an aromatic oil in its leaves and is used by some people as a flavoring. Medicinally it enjoys the reputation of being a useful remedy for respiratory ailments and chronic coughs. It can be used as a gargle for sore throats. Most modern day herbalists consider Hyssop to be effective for the lowering of blood pressure. A tea can be made of 1 oz. to 16 oz. water and taken by the wineglass — honey can be added if desired.

LEMONS
Citrus limon

How well I remember, when I was 7 years old, the family doctor calling at our house (remember those days?). He came because I had the flu and brought my mother lemons to make into barley and lemon water to help flush the kidneys. Since that time, my Mother always kept lemons in the kitchen and they became the first drink of the day, half a lemon to 8 oz. hot water. High in natural vitamin C and containing anti-infectious properties, lemons should always be available.

LICORICE ROOT
Glycyrrhiza glabra

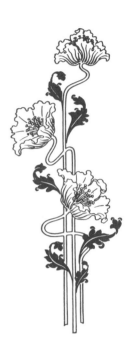

Believed to have originated in Eurasia. Licorice is widely used as a candy flavoring as well as a valuable ingredient in many pharmaceutical formulations. Considerable clinical studies have been documented on the medicinal qualities of licorice by Chinese and Western researchers alike. In western folk medicine it is considered a mild laxative, expectorant, diuretic and is used to promote healing. Generally, Herbalists consider it important for the reduction of blood cholesterol and as an antiulcer agent. It is also known to calm an upset stomach and increase the production of bile. Pharmaceutical companies use licorice in cough medicines. Singers use it to keep their throats from becoming hoarse. Roots are available from health shops.

MARJORAM
Origanum vulgare

Very familiar to Europeans as an additive to meat and poultry dishes to enhance flavor. It was used by early herbalists to aid digestion, asthma, coughs internally, and mixed with honey and applied externally as a liniment for healing of bruises. Modern day herbalists recommend it for persistent headaches and nervousness. The whole herb is medicinal and, mixed with peppermint in equal portions, acts as a general tonic. Steep 1 tsp. of the herbs to 8 oz. hot water sip slowly thoughout the day.

MELILOT
Melilotus officinalis

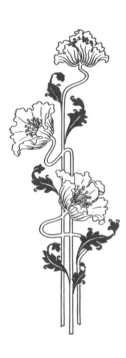

It grows freely in all areas of Britain and Europe and has a grasslike flavor. Historically it was used in the form of a poultice to treat swellings, boils and inflammations of the skin. Folk remedies treated aching rheumatic joints. It was also a tonic for the nervous system. It has mild diuretic action. Dosage 1 tsp. to 16 oz. water. Drink by the glassful.

MULLEIN LEAVES
Verbascum thapsus

If all else fails, try Mullein. This versatile herb has been used for a multitude of ills, both internal and external. It is recommended by herbalists for coughs, lung congestion and asthma. It is excellent as an expectorant and releasing phlegm congestion. Mullein leaves in vinegar and water can be used as an effective gargle for a sore throat. As a poultice for sprains and swellings it is very effective. For internal use steep 1 tsp. to 8 oz. boiling water.

MYRRH
Commiphora myrrha

Astringent, expectorant, tonic. A valuable herb believed to have originated in Arabia. It is mentioned several times in the Bible. Early herbalists used it in the treatment of ulcerated mouth and throat conditions, also as a gargle to promote healthy gums and it is considered an effective antiseptic — a tea can be made and used as a wash for hard-to-heal sores.

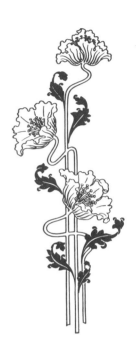

NETTLE
Urtica dioica

Used to promote the flow of urine, it is an excellent herb for kidney trouble. Also useful for colds and a fever particularly. It is a tonic for the scalp and if a tea is made (1 tsp. to 8 oz. boiling water, steep for 20 minutes) massaging it into the scalp helps to get rid of dandruff.

ONION
Allium cepa

Onions can be found in most kitchens and are usually used for culinary purposes. They are also a valuable medicine. Belonging to the lily family and esteemed by past civilizations, (Romans and Egyptians had many uses for them), the onion is used today in pharmacy for cough medicines, hay fever, etc. It is strong in sulphur compounds, very antiseptic and in

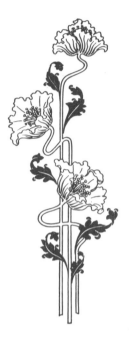

some countries like Sweden, many people eat raw onions like apples. It is claimed to be anti-aging because of its nucleic acid content. Recent studies by scientists indicate onions may be helpful for reducing cholesterol and fat content of the blood, as well as reducing hypertension.

PARSLEY
Petroselinum crispum

Cultivated as food for the Romans and medicine for the Greeks — Parsley is still regarded by herbalists as a valuable source of vitamins and minerals, particulary vitamins, A, B2, B3, C and calcium, magnesium, iron, potassium and manganese. These nutrients are readily absorbed and utilized by the body. For medicinal purposes, Parsley has been used for the prevention of kidney stones and as a tonic for the liver. It is known to dispel flatulence in the stomach and for this reason is included in many culinary recipes. Odor from the breath is eliminated by the chewing of parsley since the chlorophyll in the leaves acts as a natural deodorant. Externally for bathing the eyes, it provides relief if swollen and sore. A tea can be made by stirring 1 tsp. of leaves into 8 oz. hot water. Cool. One cup twice daily adds to general well being.

24

PEPPERMINT
Mentha piperita

Valuable menthol is extracted from peppermint. This substance is used in pharmacy to flavor medicine. Candy manufacturers and makers of toothpaste use vast quantities also as a flavoring. Its uses are numerous. It can be made into a simple tea and sipped slowly after meals for a most effective digestive aid, relieving flatulence. Peppermint grows rapidly and spreads all over the garden quickly so when planting it, take this into consideration. When dried, the leaves should be kept in airtight containers to keep their potency.

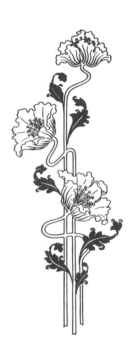

RASPBERRY LEAVES
Rubus idaeus

Mostly Raspberries are associated with delicious tasting jams and jellies. The leaves, however, have much to offer from a medicinal point of view. Both leaves and berries contain iron. One of the main ingredients of the leaves is Fragarine which strengthens the uterus of the pregnant woman. In England mid-wives give several cups of this while the mother-to-be is in labour. Good for morning sickness, for all menstruation problems such as cramping, or irregularity, excellent in preventing miscarriages. The leaves contain pectin, malic acid, calcium and potassium chloride.

RED CLOVER
Trifolium pratense

Well respected in Europe as a remedy for bronchial conditions of all kinds, modern herbalists regard it as an alterative to be used by the body to restore health generally. American Indians used it as an external remedy for burns, sores, wounds and ulcers. It can be used as a gargle to relieve a sore throat. Many European women believe it to be a safe, effective vaginal douche. It is often used to replace regular tea or coffee as an after meal beverage. A tea is made by using 2 oz. clover to 8 oz. water. For external use bathe affected parts.

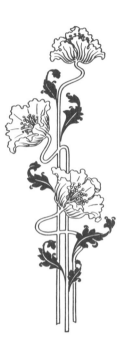

ROSE HIPS
Rosa canina

Cultivated since ancient times the rose is still considered a versatile and useful part of folk medicine. During World War II the British Government encouraged the growing of roses for the nutrient Vitamin C that could be extracted from the hips. This was used to prevent scurvy. British Scientists also discovered appreciable quantities of Vitamins A and P, which play an important role in the strengthening of capillaries and aid in the healing of wounds. Malic acid is also present in the hips and is useful for dissolving gravel from the urinary organs. Vitamin C is considered essential for the promotion of good health as well as a protection against toxic elements in the environment. As a tea it is pleasant and a good alternative to caffeine-type beverages.

ROSEMARY
Rosemarinus officinalis

Used by early herbalists to promote mental alertness and prevent fatigue, it is widely used today in the cosmetic and pharmaceutical industries. It has antiseptic qualities and is useful as a natural mouthwash for the healing of a sore throat and bleeding gums. When mixed with Mullein it is effective for bronchial conditions, especially asthma. It is rich in silicon, calcium, iron and magnesium as well as Vitamins A and C. It also is a source of protein. Rosemary is available from grocery stores and can be infused as a tea and taken by the wineglassful.

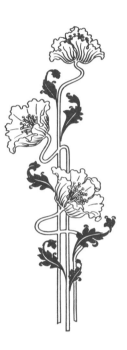

SAGE
Salvia officinalis

In modern times Sage is appreciated for its delightful aroma especially when used for culinary purposes. Early herbalists had much to say about its medicinal value and regarded it as one of the most valuable and versatile in all the plant kingdom. Considered a mild tonic, it was recommended for nervous disorders and digestive weakness. Modern herbalists recommend it when improvement of circulation is required. It is often used to treat fevers, night sweats and worms. It is also effective as a gargle. When mixed with vinegar it can be applied externally to help heal bruises.

27

THYME
Thymus vulgaris

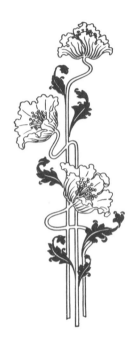

Widely cultivated in Europe and North America. It is an old favorite in folk medicine and used extensively in cosmetic and pharmaceutical products today. Early herbalists recommended it for headaches, painful menstruation, dyspepsia and to strengthen the lungs. The essential oil found in Thyme contains a powerful disinfectant called thymol that has proven effective against bacteria and fungi. It is generally used in combination with other herbs, but a tea made of 1 oz. Thyme to 16 oz. water with honey added, is an effective cold remedy. Take by the wineglassful.

VALERIAN
Valeriana officinalis

During the Middle Ages it was used for a variety of ailments, epilepsy, hysteria, insomnia, ulcers and nervous disorders. Modern day practitioners use it to calm the nervous system, promote sleep and alleviate pain. Extensive studies being conducted in European countries indicate its beneficial effects on behavioral problems in children. The odor of Valerian is not pleasant but taken as a tea with a little honey before bedtime, it promotes restful sleep.

WATERCRESS
Nasturtium officianale

28

A pungent herb used by Europeans and North American to give flavor to salads. It is a good source of nutrients such as

Vitamins A, C, E, and minerals calcium, potassium, magnesium, iron and sodium. Early settlers to America brought watercress with them as a medicine as well as a food. It was used to treat liver and kidney problems and given to the elderly to prevent hardening of the arteries. Herbalists recognize it as a blood cleanser because of its organic sulphur content. An excellent addition to sandwiches, it is found abundantly in North America in streams, springs and on nearby banks. Wash it thoroughly before eating because of possible water pollutants.

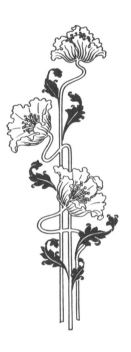

WOODRUFF
Asperula odorata

Sweet smelling and versatile, it was used to add flavor to wines and other fruit beverages. It was hung in closets as a moth repellant. Medicinally it was a mild diuretic and a tonic useful for stimulating and toning the system. Today, herbalists recommend it for liver disorders, digestive upset and externally to heal wounds and cuts.

YELLOW DOCK
Rumex crispus

Known to the Indians as a food and medicine since ancient times, it is still valuable as a mild laxative and tonic. In the 19th century it was used to heal skin eruptions such as scrofula and acne, as a blood cleanser to remove waste and as a source of natural iron. Also used externally to cleanse boils, ulcers and wounds.

COOKING WITH HERBS

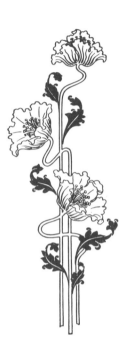

The kitchen can be described as the creation room since so many exciting, original ideas emerge from there. This is as it should be, most of us love to eat, we also enjoy new recipes or old favorites with something new added. Cooking with herbs can give you a whole new interest in taste, as well as giving health benefits along the way. It is well known that herbal seasonings induce a better flow of digestive juices, enabling us to assimilate food better. Wherever possible it is better to use the whole leaf or seeds and prepare them yourself. Prepared herbs lose a lot of their value after being ground and stored. We have no way of knowing just how old they are. When purchasing seeds and leaves, they should be kept in dark, airtight containers until ready for use. Leaves can be crushed in the hands, but seeds may need a small grinder (available at health stores). These are inexpensive and also very useful for nuts. The question most often asked is — how much should I use? One world comes to mind — sparingly! — Herbs are to enhance the flavor of foods, not disguise them. There is a general guide, depending on whether you are using fresh of dried herbs.

Suggestions

Use herbs sparingly — better to have too little than too much.

Store herbs in dark containers to protect nutrients and freshness. Painting clean jars brown will do the trick.

Remember dried herbs are two to three times stronger than fresh ones.

Dandelion leaves when young, tender and unsprayed with chemicals make a healthy substitute for lettuce. Onions and parsley added provide delightful flavor.

Save the hips of roses (after petals drop) grind in the coffee grinder. Makes a wonderful tasting tea, high in Vitamin C.

Mix your favorite herbs with flour and keep available in a dark container.

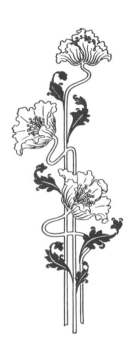

Herbs	Suggested Uses
Allspice	Pot Roast, Stews, Pickles.
Anise Seed	Cakes, Cookies, Breads, Rolls, Candies.
Balm	Teas, Fruit Drinks, Fruit Salads.
Basil	Tomato Dishes, Soups, Salads, Fish, Chicken, Cheese Dishes.
Bay Leaves	Meat, Poultry, Soups, Stews, Sauces.
Caraway Seed	Bread, Cookies, Cheeses, Cabbage Dishes, Green Salads, Vegetables.

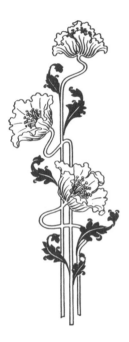

Cardamom..............Breads, Cookies,
Vegetables, Pickles.

Cayenne ....Can be used on most
foods, particularly
good with Egg Dishes.

Celery Seed...........Soups, Stews, Meats,
Poultry, Stuffings.

Chives...................Salads, Baked
Potatoes, Sauces.

Cinnamon..............Baked Goods, Stewed
Fruit, Pickles.

Cloves ....Stewed Fruit, Spiced
Drinks, Spiced Cakes,
Ham and other Meat.

Coriander Seed.......Breads, Cookies, Fruit
Sauces, Meat, Poultry,
Soups.

Cumin Seed...........Salads, Dressings,
Sauces, (Chili, Curry)
Stews.

Dill ....Vegetables, Soups,
Meats, Pickles,
Poultry, Fish.

Fennel Seed...........Cookies, Biscuits,
Candy, Jellies,
Salads, Soups, Jams.

Garlic....................Salads, Stews,
Roasts, Dressings.

Ginger...................Candies, Cookies,
Baked Goods, Stews,
Sauces, (excellent
with milk and 1
tablespoon Sesame
Tahini for energy).

Marjoram ....Meats, Poultry,
Salads, Vegetables,
Stuffings.

32

Mint......................Lamb, Peas, Salads,
Fruit Punch, Potatoes.
Nutmeg..................Cakes, Cookies,
Puddings, Custards,
Stewed Fruit.
Oregano ....Excellent for
Spaghetti, Chili,
Soups, Stuffings.
Paprika ....Vegetables, Soups,
Poultry, Meat, Fish,
gives color to bland
Egg Dishes.
Parsley...................Salads, Soups,
Vegetables, Meat,
Garnish.
Poppy Seed.............Cookies, Cakes,
Breads, Fruit Salads.
Rosemary...............Meat, Fish, Poultry,
Soups, Vegetables.
Saffron...................Fish, Poultry, Meats,
Grains (Bulgar or
Rice Dishes).
Sage......................Poultry, Fish, Meats,
Stuffings.
Summer Savory ......Soups, Bean Dishes,
Vegetables, Gravies.
Tarragon ....Salad Dressings,
Salads, Fish, Meat,
Poultry, Sauces.
Thyme...................Stuffings, Meats,
Poultry, Fish, Egg
Dishes.

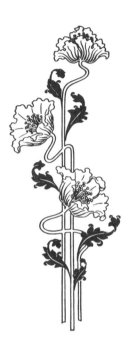

SIMPLE REMEDIES

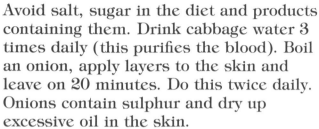

ACNE

Avoid salt, sugar in the diet and products containing them. Drink cabbage water 3 times daily (this purifies the blood). Boil an onion, apply layers to the skin and leave on 20 minutes. Do this twice daily. Onions contain sulphur and dry up excessive oil in the skin.

Steam the skin 3 times a week with Anise Seed (1 tablespoon to a bowl of water).

Drink fresh vegetable juices, especially carrot and celery.

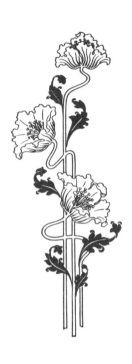

ANEMIA

Old-fashioned remedies for anemia were usually made up in the kitchen and given as part of the daily diet. The following remedies are all rich in natural iron.

1. **Tonic**
   1 cup tomato juice
   4 oz. water
   juice of ½ lemon
   1 stalk of celery
   2 oz. diced calve's liver
   Put all ingredients into the blender and liquify for 2 minutes. Serves 2.
2. Yellow Dock, Yarrow, Wild Cherry Bark, Comfrey, Red Raspberry. A simple tea can be made 2 or 3 times daily of either of the above herbs.
3. 1 tbsp. Blackstrap Molasses in 8 oz. hot water each morning first thing.

4. Eating berries of all kinds (raw, not in pies). Blackberries, Black Currants, Blueberries, Cranberries, Red Currants, Grapes.
5. 1 cup leaves of spinach, 4 sticks celery, 1 carrot, half a tomato. Blend altogether. Excellent blood builder.

ARTHRITIS

Many sufferers from Arthritis have used the following with varying results and most agree that they feel better when they:
1. Drink 3 or 4 cups of Alfalfa tea daily.
2. Take Epsom's Salt baths.
3. Eat Celery and Parsley.
4. Drink the juice of Cucumbers, matched with equal amounts unsweetened Pineapple juice and half a Lime. Blend altogether. This mixture is to dissolve caculi in the joints.
5. Use Sunflower Seeds and Cod Liver Oil for the vitamin A content.
6. Drink Willow Bark tea. This herb contains Salicyn — (used as a pain killer). 1 cup daily is recommended.
7. Get rid of acid wastes in the body by building a strong alkaline reserve. Eat mainly alkaline foods.

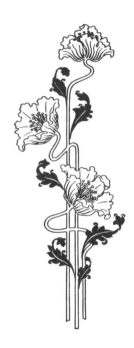

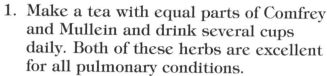

ASTHMA

1. Make a tea with equal parts of Comfrey and Mullein and drink several cups daily. Both of these herbs are excellent for all pulmonary conditions.
2. Drink Garlic juice (2 Cloves), mixed with a little pure, unpasteurized honey and take several times daily, or drink garlic tea made with fresh cloves or oil of garlic.
3. An alkaline diet (mainly fruits, vegetables, raw seeds, Sunflower, Sesame, Flax, Almonds). Stay away from dairy products and mucous-forming foods.

ATHLETE'S FOOT

1. Squeeze the pulp of Aloe Vera plant directly onto affected area several times daily.
2. Dab on Apple Cider Vinegar undiluted.
3. Slice of raw Onion applied directly.

BACKACHE (Due to Kidneys)

Make a tea with Juniper Berries or Buchu leaves and drink 3 or 4 cups daily.

Juice of half a lemon in 8 oz. warm water, morning and night. Watermelon juice taken freely is excellent.

36

BITES — (Insects)

1. For stings and bites, mix together 1 oz. Chamomile, 1 oz. Nettle leaves, 1 oz. Sage, 1 cup boiling water. Pour water onto herbs, let steep 15 minutes covered, add 1 tsp. lemon juice, strain and apply directly.
2. Take a slice of raw lemon and apply.
3. Apply a drop or two or Echinacea tincture.

BLADDER

Barley and lemon water, according to grandma, is supposed to be good for the waterworks. Add 4 oz. barley to 32 oz. water. When cooked remove from heat and strain. To the water add the juice of a lemon. Sip throughout the day.

Cranberry juice (sugarless) has been used with great success for cystitis.

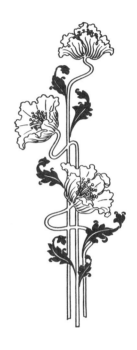

BLOOD PRESSURE — High

Sliver 1 clove Garlic into 1 oz. milk before retiring at night and drink. Nettle tea can also be taken several times daily.

BOILS

Boil an Onion and apply a slice, warm, directly onto affected area. Repeat several times daily.

BRONCHIAL PROBLEMS

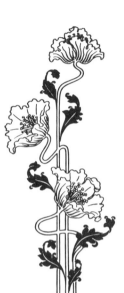

1. When there is an excess of mucous, take two lemons, cut in half, put honey between and bake at 350 degrees Farhenheit, for three quarters of an hour. Scrape out pulp and eat. (This cuts congestion).
2. Drink freely of Comfrey, Mullein, Lungwort tea.
3. Cut up raw Onion, sprinkle on honey and leave overnight. A liquid will form, this can be taken by the tsp. several times daily.
4. Pine needles added to the bathwater are very beneficial. Relieves congestion.
5. Squeeze garlic clove into 8 oz. hot water. Sip slowly.

BRUISES

1. Immerse affected part in hot water for 15 minutes.
2. Make a tea with 1 tsp. Mullein leaves to 8 oz. water, strain and place leaves in cotton gauze. Apply to bruise.
3. Apply pressure to bruise. Halts internal bleeding.
4. Raw potato thinly sliced, apply to bruise and cover, change often.
5. Adequate vitamin C prevents bruising.

BURNS

1. Take a Comfrey leaf, smear with unpasteurized honey and apply to burn, cover with gauze, change daily.
2. Peel back Aloe Vera leaf, squeeze gel directly onto burn.
3. Put affected part into cold water, leave until pain has gone, then apply scraped raw potato.
4. Apply white of egg.

CALLOUSES & CORNS

Take a slice of raw lemon, place over affected area. Tape in place and leave on overnight. Raw onion can also be used in this manner. Use olive oil to soften, then lift out corn.

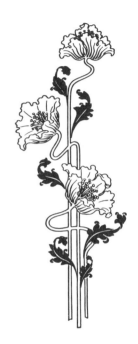

CANKER SORES

Dab on pure honey, let dissolve on sore.

CARBUNCLE

Mix an egg yolk with a pinch of salt — apply to carbuncle. Cover with gauze.

CHILLBLAINS

1. Use own urine, dab directly onto affected area. Soothes itchiness.
2. Bath with warm salt water.

CIRCULATION

Take 1 inch of fresh ginger root, grate into 8 oz. hot water. Sip slowly.

COLD HANDS & FEET

1. Take 1/10 tsp. of Cayenne Pepper in 1 glass water. This steps up circulation and provides warmth.
2. For warm feet, sprinkle Cayenne sparingly in shoes or boots. (Especially beneficial for ski fans).

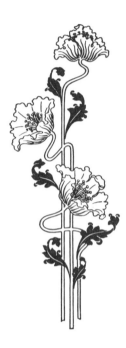

COLIC

Make a tea of Chamomile. 1 tbsp. to 1 pint boiling water and give a tsp. to colicky baby, 3 or 4 times daily.

CONSTIPATION

Millions of dollars are spent annually on laxatives. It is probably the number one health problem of the North American Continent. Bulk and fiber is needed in the diet to produce healthy bowel movements, plus a fair amount of water to flush the system. If you do allow yourself to become constipated, listed below are several natural and inexpensive remedies.

1. 1 tbsp. of Molasses in 8 oz. warm water and juice of half a lemon first thing in the morning.
2. 1 tbsp. Flaxseed in 2 tbsp. warm water. Allow to stand all night, it becomes soft and jelly like. Swallow first thing in the morning.

40

3. 1 cup Senna tea with a pinch of Ginger (this prevents cramping) taken before bedtime.
4. Eat 3 figs slowly, first thing in the morning, followed by a glass of warm water 1 hour later.
5. Make a cereal of the following:
   1 tbsp. of Flaxseed Meal
   1 cup cold water
   1 tbsp. vinegar
   ½ tsp. honey.
   Bring to near boiling, cool and eat.
   Don't forget to exercise.

COUGH & COLDS

1. Make a tea of any of the following: Garlic, Horehound, Comfrey. Do not drink any milk but only fruit juices or herb teas, (as directed).
2. Suck slowly on a piece of Honeycomb. (Relieves cough.)
3. Onions and Honey. (See Bronchial problems.)
4. Mix together equal parts of Peppermint and Elder flowers, make a tea and drink 3 or 4 cups daily. (This breaks up a cold.)
5. Before retiring, drink Sage tea, soak feet in a mustard bath and inhale fumes. (3 tbsp. of dry mustard in enough water to cover ankles.) Then put on warm socks, wrap up well and keep covered in bed. This induces perspiration and clears the system of mucous.

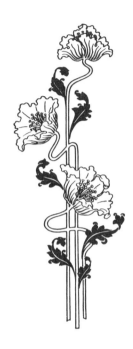

41

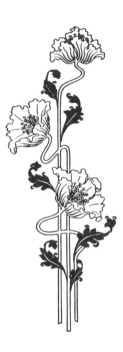

6. Make a tea with 1 tsp. Thyme to 8 oz. hot water. Substitute for a regular beverage.
7. Grate a little Horseradish into a cup of hot water. Add honey to taste.
8. Make your favorite chicken noodle soup — then add 1 oz. freshly grated ginger root to it.

CRADLE CAP

Warm Olive Oil, take a Q-Tip and apply gently all over the scalp. The crust will lift after the oil has soaked in.

CRAMPS

1. Stomach cramps can be helped with the use of grated ginger root in warm water. 1 inch of root to 8 oz. water, sip slowly.
2. Chew anise seeds thoroughly for stomach cramps.
3. Menstrual Cramps have been known to disappear with the sipping of Fennel Seed tea made with 1 tsp. crushed seeds to 8 oz. hot water.
4. 1 oz. dried parsley leaves to 1 quart of boiling water. Let cool, strain and sip throughout the day. This was grandma's remedy for menstrual cramps.
5. Leg cramps can be relieved by gently massaging along the calf muscles toward the heart. This increases circulation.

42

CROUP

See Bronchial No. 3

CUTS

Apply unpasteurized honey to cut and cover, heals quickly.

DANDRUFF

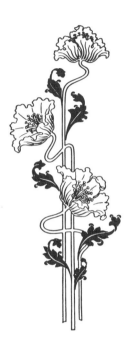

1. Take the juice of Aloe Vera plant, massage into the scalp. Apply hot wet towel and leave on 20 minutes. Shampoo with mild shampoo and have a final rinse with Apple Cider Vinegar, (½ cup to last rinse water). Do this twice weekly.
2. Add 1 oz. sulphur to 32 oz. water, wash the scalp once daily with this solution until clear.
3. A strong solution of salt water massaged into the scalp every other day alternated with a massage of warm olive oil.
4. Mix 1 tbsp. nettle leaves with 8 oz. apple cider vinegar and bring to a boil. Cool and massage into scalp.

DIAPER RASH

Put 1½ cups oatmeal in tub, put enough water to cover and sit child in it for 20 minutes. Do this morning and night.

DIARRHEA

1. Drink apple juice liberally sprinkled with cinnamon.
2. Make a mild tea of Strawberry leaves and drink freely.

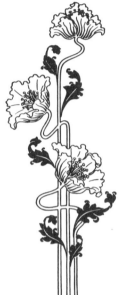

DIGESTION

Choice of the following:
1. 1 tbsp. undiluted Papaya Juice, half an hour after meals.
2. 1 cup Peppermint tea, half an hour after meals. Anise Seeds can be used in the same manner. Use 1 tsp. leaves to 1 cup boiling water.
3. Eat sprig of Parsley after meals.
4. 1 tsp. of Olive Oil taken before or with meals.
5. Eliminate drinking water with meals. No liquid should be taken until at least half an hour after.

EARACHE

1. Boil an Onion until soft, take out the center core and insert into the ear canal. Garlic clove also works (uncooked). Be careful not to push into the ear canal too far.
2. Warm Olive Oil, drop into the ear, then apply a warm salt bag. (Make a cotton bag, fill with salt and heat in the oven). Brings instant relief. The bag could be made ahead of time — and kept for emergencies.

ECZEMA

1. Mix equal amounts of Cider Vinegar and water. Dab on affected area several times daily.
2. 1 tbsp. lecithin granules taken daily (sprinkle on cereals or blend in juices). Beet, celery and tomato juice are beneficial for all skin problems.
3. Boil together 1 oz. Burdock Root to 1½ pints water until approximately 1 pint is left. Drink 1 oz. 3 times daily.
4. Place 4 oz. vaseline and 4 oz. pure lanolin in baking dish, add 4 oz. Chickweed, cook in oven 325 degrees Farhenheit until herbs strain through a clean cheesecloth. Use mixture on Eczema.
5. Take internally, 1 tbsp. of Safflower Oil twice a day — have plenty of B vitamin foods.

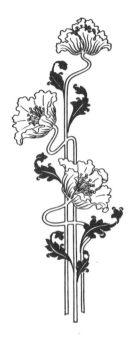

FEET (sore)

Put 8 oz. salt into a footbath. Add water to cover ankles and soak for 20 minutes.

Feet ache? Put under hot running water for a few minutes, then cold. Repeat. Swollen feet can be helped by immersing them in hot water then cold. Repeat several times.

FELON

1. Tie a piece of lemon to affected area — leave on overnight.
2. If you pinch a finger — hold in cold water until pain leaves.

45

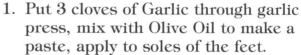

FEVERS

1. Put 3 cloves of Garlic through garlic press, mix with Olive Oil to make a paste, apply to soles of the feet.
2. Wash down body with tepid water to which as been added half a cup Apple Cider Vinegar.
3. Drink fruit juices of all kinds (no dairy).

FLATULENCE

(See Digestion).

FRECKLES

1. Slice a lemon and rub gently over freckled area. This helps to bleach freckles but only on a temporary basis. Direct sunlight will encourage freckles to return. Be sure to use moisture after this treatment as lemon tends to dry the skin.
2. Buttermilk applied 3 times daily helps to bleach freckles.

GOUT

Mix equal amounts of carrot and celery juice, throw in some alfalfa — drink 2 oz. 6 times daily.

When the pain becomes unbearable — take internally , a tea made with endive (boil together 1 tbsp. to 1 pint water) — let cool. Drink a cup, this greatly alleviates the pain.

Make a poultice of bran — put into a cheesecloth and apply to affected part.

GUMS (to strengthen)

1. ½ tsp. salt in 8 oz. water, swish through teeth and around gums. Do this often.

HAIR

1. Aloe Vera Gel massaged into the scalp, then a hot, wet, towel wrapped around for 15 minutes, conditions and strengthens hair.
2. Take warm Olive Oil, massage into scalp, apply hot, wet towel. Leave on 30 minutes — shampoo well, this is especially good for dry, brittle hair.

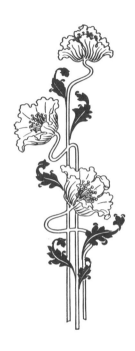

HAYFEVER

1. Mix 3 drops each of the following: Peppermint Oil, Oil of Cloves, Oil of Rosemary, inhale as needed.
2. Fill the hollow of the hand with Witchhazel and inhale deeply, repeat as necessary.

HEARTBURN

1. Make a simple tea with Fennel Seeds, let steep, strain and sip slowly. Ginger tea is also effective.
2. 1 tsp. of Apple Cider Vinegar in 4 oz. water. Sip slowly.

HEMORRHOID

1. Peel back an Aloe Vera leaf and take out some of the gel. Insert into the rectum. Change dressing several times daily.
2. Make a poultice of roasted Onions, apply directly.
3. Make a Comfrey tea, let it get cold, use a cotton swab to bathe the area several times daily.
4. Apply a piece of ice to the area, this will contract the veins and bring welcome relief. Hold in place with small towel.
5. Insert small piece of cocoa butter each evening into rectum, leave to melt overnight.
6. Omit from the diet, alcohol, spiced foods, white flour and sugar products.

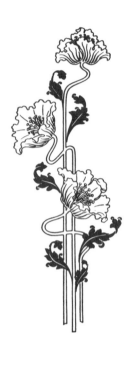

HICCUPS

1. Use 1 tsp. fennel seeds to 1 cup boiling water. Sip slowly.
2. 4 oz. hot water with ¼ tsp. ginger.

INSOMNIA

1. Eat celery 1 hour before retiring.
2. Make a nightcap of Hop tea, 1 tsp. to 1 cup of boiling water, let steep then sip slowly. Comfrey tea is also helpful because of its calcium content. (Calcium relaxes).

3. Stand in front of an open window, breathe in slowly and deeply to the count of 7, exhale to the same count. Do this several times.

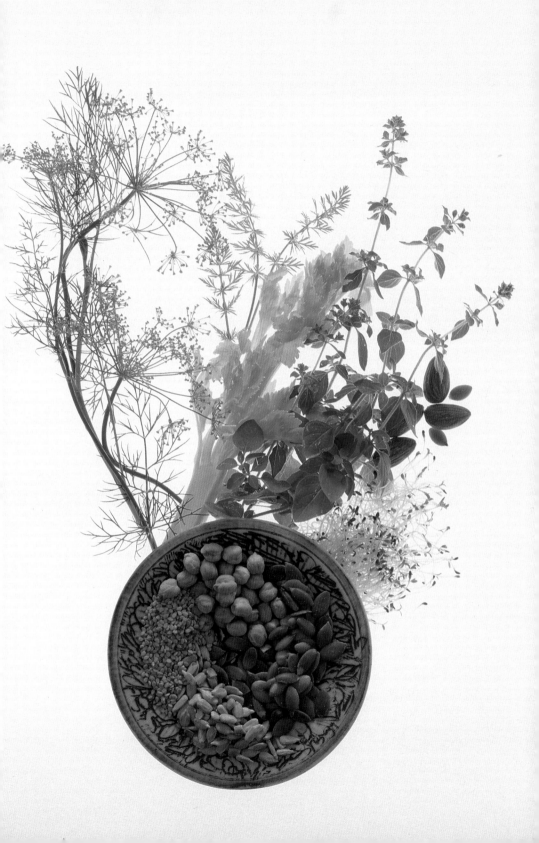

A WORD ABOUT FOODS
Almonds
Alfalfa Sprouts
Pumpkin Seeds
Sunflower Seeds
Sesame Seeds
Garbanzo Beans
Dill
Celery
Oregano
Caraway

4. One pinch of nutmeg in an 8 oz. glass of warm milk — sip slowly.
5. Bathe feet in hot water before retiring — very relaxing.
6. 1 cup onion soup an hour before retiring.

KIDNEYS

1. To keep kidneys in healthy condition, the following recipe helps to dissolve stones.
   Mix together: —
       8 oz. carrot juice,
       4 oz. beet juice,
       4 oz. cucumber juice.
   Take 1 glass 3 times daily.
2. Upon arising each morning, the juice of ½ lemon in 8 oz. warm water (a dash of molasses is delicious and keeps bowels open).
3. Drink 3 glasses cranberry juice daily.
4. Boil crushed Watermelon Seeds, strain then give 2 tbsp. every ½ hour.

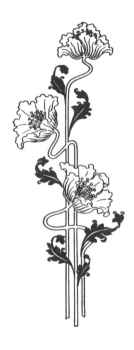

LUMBAGO

Drink celery juice mixed with a little carrot for a sweeter taste.

Make a poultice with hot bran and apply moist to affected part. Rest in bed. A mustard plaster is also helpful as an alternative.

49

MENOPAUSE

1. This is a time of hormone change in the body. Black Cohosh is excellent for normalizing. This can be taken in tablet form or as a tea.
2. Dang Quai seems to help any condition with relation to female glands, i.e.: irregular menstruation and helps to control hot flushes. This herb can be found in herb shops and can be taken as tea or in capsules.

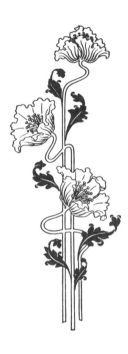

MENSTRUATION

See above. Also see CRAMPS.

1. Calcium tablets taken a week before period is due (at least 6 a day seems to relieve cramping). Drink Comfrey tea for natural calcium.
2. Raspberry leaf tea taken 3 times daily strengthens female organs.
3. To increase flow, Penny Royal herb can be taken, ½ tsp. to 8 oz. boiling water.
4. To decrease flow, take 1 tsp. gelatin in juice daily.

MIGRAINE

1. Take a hot footbath, soak a towel in cold Apple Cider Vinegar and apply to forehead. Sip on hot peppermint tea. (Massage area gently just below rib cage on the left side of the body).
2. Eat an orange.

MONONUCLEOSIS

1. Drink several cups of Raspberry Leaf tea each day.
2. Take Garlic daily to help cleanse bloodstream, drink lots of fresh fruit juices.

NOSEBLEED

Insert finger coated with vaseline directly into nostrils.

Cold compresses to the back of the neck.

NURSING HINTS

4 oz. Alfalfa tea twice daily helps to increase milk supply.

For softening breast during nursing gently bathe with parsley tea.

PINWORMS

1. Peel a clove of Garlic, hold under the tongue and let dissolve. Do not eat. Do this for 1 whole day. Replace clove as needed.
2. Raw Pumpkin seeds chewed slowly with no other food for 1 day is also effective.

POISON IVY

Cut up 1 Onion, pour over 8 oz. boilng water, cool and apply with cotton to affected part.

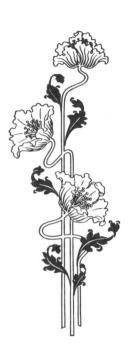

PROSTATE

1. Eat a handful of raw Pumpkin seeds daily. These seeds are high in zinc.
2. Ginseng is an excellent herb for the glands, which can be taken as powder or in liquid form. Many people have had excellent results from the use of this plant.

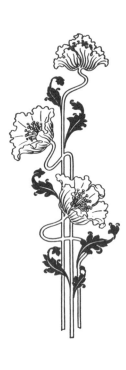

RHEUMATISM

1. Add ½ oz. sage to 12 oz. boiling water. Let sit for 15 minutes. Drink 4 oz. at a time.
2. A sprinkle of cayenne pepper in a cup of hot water brings warmth and increased circulation.
3. Celery juice is also beneficial, especially if mixed with a little carrot juice. At least 2 glasses a day should be taken.
4. Cayenne pepper brings warmth to the body and improves the circulation. This seems helpful in rheumatism.

Externally

1. A mustard plaster generates heat to the affected area.
2. Eucalyptus and wintergreen oils massaged into stiff areas bring relief.

SHINGLES

Stress is a contributing factor to shingles. Eating foods with a high content of the B vitamins plus vitamin C is very helpful. Calcium & magnesium have a calming effect on nerves also. Comfrey leaves have an abundance of both.

SINUS CONDITION

A little grated horseradish root in hot water can be taken by the teaspoonful.

SORE THROAT

1. Gargle with 1 tbsp. of Apple Cider Vinegar in 8 oz. water. Make a tea with Garlic and sip slowly throughout the day. (2 cloves to 1 pint of water).
2. The juice of ½ lemon in 8 oz. hot water gives good vitamin C content. Take at least 2 cups daily.
3. Chew on Licorice Root stick (found in health stores).
4. Salt water gargle.
5. Sage tea is an old standby, 1 oz. sage to 16 oz. boiling water. Let sit 10 minutes. Strain, use as gargle.

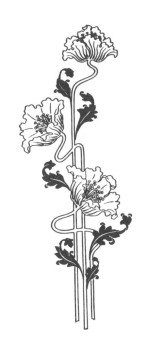

SPRAINS

1. Mix white of an egg, add salt to mixture until a paste is formed, apply to sprain.
2. Comfrey leaves dampened and applied to area bring relief.

STYE

1. Shred a raw potato, apply directly to eye, this helps to heal.
2. A gold ring rubbed on the stye several times daily.

SUNBURN (See burns also)

1. 1 tbsp. Witch hazel extract, white of 1 egg, ¼ tsp. of honey beat together and apply to burn.
2. Aloe Vera applied directly from plant takes pain away immediately.
3. To prevent sunburn, apply sesame oil to body 1 hour before going into the sun. This way the skin does not dry. Most effective lotions contain a sun screen PABA, which are available at health food stores.

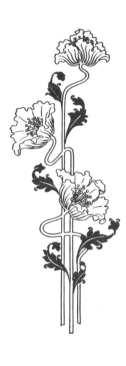

TOOTHACHE

Oil of Cloves or a whole Clove inserted into the cavity.

ULCERS

Cabbage and carrot juice contain vitamin U, plus vitamins A and C. These are valuable in healing stomach ulcers. The amounts should be as follows: ⅔ carrot to ⅓ cabbage juice, 6 glasses daily for 6 days. When followed faithfully, the results are remarkable. Most ulcer diets are bland and meant merely to coat the ulcer; this juice remedy actually heals it.

VAGINAL ITCH

Douche with a mild tea of Chamomile flowers. This remedy is used by Russian women as a preventive measure against this problem.

54

VARICOSE VEINS

1. Apply ice to the affected area with a towel. This helps to contract veins.
2. Apply Witch Hazel morning and night.
3. Vitamin E taken internally has produced good results.

WARTS

1. Dab on Milkweed several times daily.
2. Vitamin E applied directly has produced good results in some people.
3. Raw Onion Juice applied morning and night.

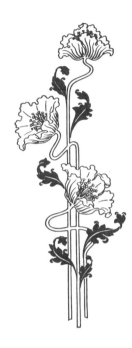

WEIGHT CONTROL

1. This seems more a case of what not to do more than what to do. However, there are certain herbs that help to lose weight. Bladderwrack is one of them, make a simple tea and take 4 oz. 3 times daily.
2. 3 Kelp tablets taken ½ hour before meals also helps.
3. Chewing gum can put on weight (even sugarless), the action of chewing stimulates the saliva and the stomach prepares to digest making the gum chewer hungry, thus more food than necessary is usually consumed.
4. Eliminating liquids with meals has the same effect as above.

55

WRINKLES

See Beauty Section.

VITAMINS

Since Vitamins and Minerals play such a large part in keeping our bodies healthy, this portion of the book is devoted to Vitamin and Mineral deficiencies and how to correct them through choosing the right foods. Herbs are also included as these supply an inexpensive way of obtaining valuable nutrients.

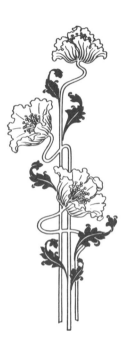

VITAMIN A

This Vitamin is measured in units. It is fat soluble which means it is found most abundantly in fatty foods. It is stored in the liver by the body (which is why the highest amounts of Vitamin A are found in halibut and cod liver oil). It is essential for building resistance to infection, promotes growth and is espcially beneficial for the skin. It is known for counteracting night-blindness and weakness in the eyes. There is indication that television and fluorescent lights may deplete the body of this Vitamin.

DEFICIENCY SYMPTOMS

Incrased susceptability to infection, frequent colds, night-blindness, dry skin, poor nails, lack of appetite, allergies, itching and burning eyes, soft teeth enamel.

FOOD SOURCES

Carrots, Spinach, Green leafy vegetables, Dairy products, Beet greens, Dandelion Greens, Pumpkin, Almonds, Fish liver oils, Figs, Apples, Cucumber, Banana, Comfrey, Celery, Alfalfa, Parsley, Red Clover, Dandelion.

VITAMIN B.1 (Thiamine)

Water soluble and much like Vitamin A, B.1 is essential for growth, for the nervous system and aids in digestion.

DEFICIENCY SYMPTOMS

Digestive disturbances, irritability, shortness of breath, depression, loss of appetite, constipation.

FOOD SOURCES

Wheat Germ, Brewer's Yeast, Blackstrap Molasses, Whole Grains, Nuts, Vegetables, Watermelon, Lemons, Grapefruit, Blackberries, Bananas, Cherries, Peaches, Bladderwrack, Parsley.

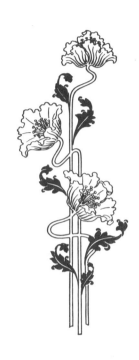

VITAMIN B.2 (Riboflavin)

Promotes general health, good vision, healthy skin and aids the intestinal tract.

DEFICIENCY SYMPTOMS

Poor disgestion, liver spots, dizziness, itching and burning eyes, wrinkles around the lips, sore tongue, bloodshot eyes.

FOOD SOURCES

Brewer's Yeast, Blackstrap Molasses, Wheat Germ, Poultry, Fish, Milk, Pumpkin Seeds, Sunflower Seeds, Comfrey leaves, Celery, Bladderwrack.

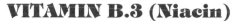

VITAMIN B.3 (Niacin)

Important for the nervous system, maintains normal function of the intestinal tract. When taken in tablet form, Niacin brings the blood to the surface of the skin increasing circulation and causing a prickly sensation in some people. It has been used with great success for hyperactive children, alcoholism, circulatory problems, mental weakness.

DEFICIENCY SYMPTOMS

Mental depression, vague aches and pains, loss of appetite and general weakness.

FOOD SOURCES

Brewer's Yeast, Rice Polishings, Green Vegetables, Wheat Germ, Nuts, (especially Sunflower Seeds, Alfalfa, Fenugreek, Parsley.)

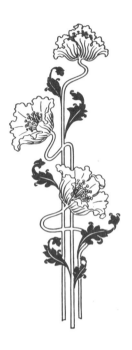

VITAMIN B.6 (Pyridoxine)

This Vitamin has been popular in recent years because of its effectiveness against water retention, therefore helping with weight problems. It is an aid for food assimilation, nausea, and again for treatment of depression.

DEFICIENCY SYMPTOMS

Irritability, skin erruptions, lack of muscular control, anemia, constant tiredness.

FOOD SOURCES

Wheat Germ, Egg Yolk, Brewer's Yeast, Green Leafy Vegetables, Wholegrain Cereals, Organ Meats, Comfrey.

VITAMIN B.12 (Cabolomin)

Very beneficial for anemia, helps in the regeneration of red blood cells, promotes growth, aids nervous conditions, especially depression.

DEFICIENCY SYMPTOMS

Constantly tired, poor appetite, loss of mental energy, general run down feeling, fear, anemia.

FOOD SOURCES

Organ meats, Fish, Cheese, Brewer's Yeast, Wheat Germ, Nuts, Grapes, Raspberries, and Strawberries, Comfrey leaves.

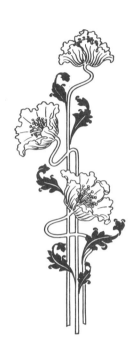

VITAMIN B.15 (Panagamic Acid)

Helps to regulate fat metabolism, stimulates the nervous system, circulation. Much has been written on it concerning premature aging, useful in treating weak muscles.

DEFICIENCY SYMPTOMS

May cause glandular and nervous disorders.

FOOD SOURCES
Wholegrain Cereals, Nuts, Seeds, Rice Bran.

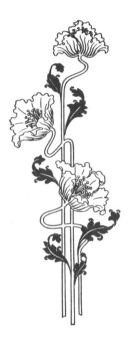

VITAMIN B.17 (Laetrille)
There is much controversy over this Vitamin. Clinics in Mexico are using it to treat malignancies. Some members of the medical profession in Canada and the United States claim it is useless, others believe it has some value. The food sources of this Vitamin include the seeds of Apricots, Apple, Buckwheat and Flaxseed.

OTHER MEMBERS OF B. COMPLEX

PANTOTHENIC ACID
Known to be helpful in the building of body cells, maintaining normal skin growth and helpful for the digestive processes. All the functions of Pantothenic Acid have not been defined as yet.

DEFICIENCY SYMPTOMS
Painful and burning feet, digestive disturbances, irritability, muscular weakness.

FOOD SOURCES
Kidney, Liver, Egg Yolks, Brewer's Yeast, Wheat Germ, Bran.

P.A.B.A.
(para-Amino Benzoic Acid)

Needed for promoting growth, helpful for skin, used in the treatment of gray hair.

DEFICIENCY SYMPTOMS

Anemia, extreme tiredness.

FOOD SOURCES

Wholegrains, Wheat Germ, Brewer's Yeast, Eggs, Liver.

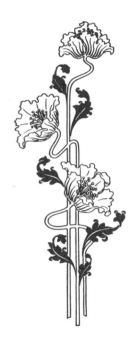

CHOLINE

One of the lipotropic factors necessary for normal fat metabolism, also regulates the function of the liver.

DEFICIENCY SYMPTOMS

May result in hardening of the arteries, degeneration of the liver.

FOOD SOURCES

Fruits of all kinds, Almonds, Sunflower Seeds, Whole Grains, Brewer's Yeast, Liver, Wheat Germ.

FOLIC ACID

Helps in formation of red blood cells, aids protein metabolism and contributes to normal growth, helpful in hair growth.

DEFICIENCY SYMPTOMS

61

Skin disorders, mental depression, may lead to hair loss.

FOOD SOURCES

Organ meats, Brewer's Yeast, Wheat
Germ, Nuts, Green Leafy Vegetables.

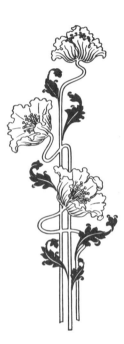

BIOTIN

Especially good for promoting growth,
especially the hair.

DEFICIENCY SYMPTOMS

General fatigue, skin disorders.

FOOD SOURCES

Brewer's Yeast, Liver, Soybeans,
Sunflower Seeds.

VITAMIN C

Necessary for healthy teeth, gums, bones,
strengthens all connective tissue,
promotes healing of wounds, acts as a
detoxifier and cleans the system generally.

DEFICIENCY SYMPTOMS

Anemia, gum disorders, bruise easily,
cavities, low cold resistance, capillary
weakness, loss of appetite.

FOOD SOURCES

Citrus Fruits, Berries, Cantaloupe, Green
Peppers, Cabbage, Tomatoes, Rosehips,
Malvah Blossoms, Parsley, Alfalfa.

VITAMIN D

Regulates the use of Calcium and Phosphorous in the body. Necessary for the proper formation of teeth and bones.

DEFICIENCY SYMPTOMS

May lead to rickets, tooth decay, retarded growth, muscular weakness, diarrhea, insomnia.

FOOD SOURCES

Egg Yolks, Milk, Butter, Bonemeal, Fish, Organ Meats, Alfalfa Sprouts, Cress, Garlic.

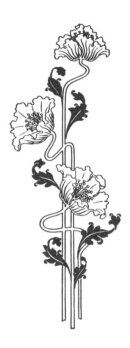

VITAMIN E

Is probably one of the most popular Vitamins sold. Many claims have been made for Vitamin E, but Dr. Shute of London, Ontario, used it with great success for the prevention of heart disease, burns, leg ulcers, varicose veins, etc. Since then it has been used for general well being, sterility, and the healing of skin problems. Research has not been completed as yet, but people taking Vitamin E claim they feel more energetic.

DEFICIENCY SYMPTOMS

May lead to strokes and heart disease. Enlarged prostate, impotency, dry dull hair.

FOOD SOURCES

Vegetable Oils, Whole-Grain Cereals, Sunflower Seeds, Eggs, Wheat Germ, Organ Meats, Green Vegetables, Alfalfa, Linseed, Cress, Parsley.

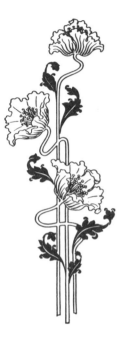

VITAMIN K

Aids in blood clotting.

DEFICIENCY SYMPTOMS

Hemorrhages resulting from prolonged blood clotting time.

FOOD SOURCES

Egg Yolks, Soybean Oil, Alfalfa.

MINERALS

Adequate Minerals are just as essential to the body as Vitamins. They do, in fact, work closely together. Every cell in the body contains small amounts of almost all the Mineral elements; however, Calcium and Phosphorous are the dominating Minerals due to the skeletal framework, the bulk of which is made up of these elements.

CALCIUM

As well as being an essential element for building bone, it is also necessary for the normal clotting of blood. Many people who have studied Adelle Davis' excellent book "Let's Eat Right to Keep Fit" claim that by eating Calcium-rich foods, or by taking extra supplementation, they feel more stable emotionally, sleep better and have less muscle cramps. An adequate supply of calcium calms the nervous system and promotes a general sense of well being.

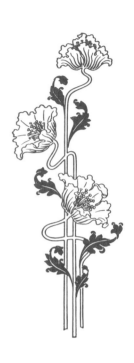

DEFICIENCY SYMPTOMS

May cause irritability, poor teeth, muscle cramps, insomnia, fragile bones.

FOOD SOURCES

Bonemeal, Milk, Egg Yolk, Cheese, Nuts, Green Vegetables, Dandelion Greens, Chard, Soybeans, Celery, Oranges, Strawberries, Raspberries, Prunes, Comfrey Leaves, Coltsfoot, Chamomile, Blackstrap Molasses, Figs, Watercress, Broccoli, Olives.

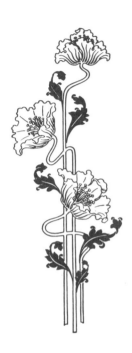

COPPER

Works very closely with Iron. It is a trace mineral and our bodies require small amounts. The function of this element appears to be associated with Iron in producing hemoglobin. There is an excellent chapter on Copper in J. Rodale's book "The Health Builder". He warns of the use of cooking with copper utensils because of the danger of copper poisoning. He advises against the use of water from the hot pipes if they are copper. There is a difference, of course, in Copper from food sources.

DEFICIENCY SYMPTOMS

May lead to anemia, impaired respiratory, digestive problems.

FOOD SOURCES

Whole-Grain Products, Beans, Molasses, Liver, Fish, Nuts.

IODINE

Is needed by the thyroid glands to produce a hormone known as thyroxin, which, in turn, affects general development, mental and physical. Iodine deficiency can cause an enlargement of the thyroid glands commonly called goiter. The problem is more common than it should be. People who have problems with body temperature i.e. cold extremities or are unable to control body weight or have a general sluggish feeling with mental fatigue should check out the Thyroid glands.

DEFICIENCY SYMPTOMS

Can cause goiter, overweight, general fatigue, irritability.

FOOD SOURCES

Seafoods of all kinds, Cod Liver Oil, Swiss Chard, Asparagus, Kelp.

IRON

Necessary for hemoglobin — the red pigment of blood cells. These blood cells travel around the body carrying oxygen, without which we could not live. Iron, then, is of vital importance in supplying the body with life-oxygen. Anyone who has suffered from Iron deficiency can tell of the fatigue, depression, irritability and shortness of breath. Women need an abundance of Iron due to the loss during menstruation. Children also need a good supply since they grow so rapidly. Many people take Iron supplements, but for some reason, these can cause constipation and do not live up to their advertising claims. Iron-rich foods are the best sources. Nature is an excellent chemist and prepares the balance needed by the body for better assimilation.

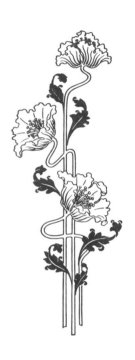

DEFICIENCY SYMPTOMS

May lead to anemia, headaches, fatigue, irritability, overall general weakness.

FOOD SOURCES

67

Egg Yolks, Liver, Kidney, Dried Apricots, Figs, Dried Prunes, Raisins, Dates,

Molasses, Walnuts, Peanuts, Whole Wheat, Oysters, Beet Tops, Chard, Watercress, Parsley, Dandelion Greens, Spinach, Cabbage, Broccoli, Burdock Root, Nettle Leaves.

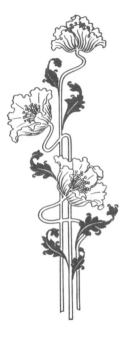

MAGNESIUM

This is important in relation to the utilization of Calcium as well as other minerals. The main source of this element is in green vegetables and whole grains. Unfortunately, once the whole grain is refined, much of the Magnesium is removed. Magnesium is necessary for healthy nerves and normal functioning of the muscular system. It also aids digestion and general circulation.

DEFICIENCY SYMPTOMS

May lead to muscle cramps, irritability, depression and kidney stones.

FOOD SOURCES

Whole Grains (Wheat, Brown Rice, Barley, Corn, Oats), Nuts (Sesame Seeds, Almonds, Brazil Nuts, Pecans, Walnuts), Parsley, Watercress, Corn Silk, Walnut Leaves, Mullein, Potatoes, Brewer's Yeast.

PHOSPHORUS

We do not know exactly all of the functions of this Mineral; however, we do know it works closely with Calcium and is found in bones and teeth for the most part, but is also found in the muscles and nerves in the rest of the body. Phosphorus is found in most foods so it is hard to imagine anyone having a deficiency. It is, however, tied in so closely with Calcium that balance is necessary to provide the body with its needs. Therefore, added bonemeal taken as a supplement would give some nutritional insurance.

DEFICIENCY SYMPTOMS

May cause general weakness of nerves and mental ability. Also retarded growth.

FOOD SOURCES

Egg Yolks, Cheese, Milk, Almonds, Peanuts, Hazelnuts, Walnuts, Pecans, Raisins, Brussels Sprouts, Apricots, Figs, Fresh Corn, Prunes, Parsnips, Broccoli, Whole Grains, Watercress, Chickweed, Meadow sweet.

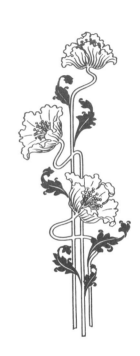

POTASSIUM

This element is required to regulate the balance of body fluids. It is also present in the network that makes up the skin and red blood cells. It is needed for normal growth, muscle function and helps with the working of the digestive tract. Potassium is found in a great many foods. It has to have balance in the system with Sodium, for there is evidence that too much Sodium can cause an imbalance. This is one reason we have to be careful about adding salt to everything we eat. Rodale has an excellent chapter on this in "The Health Builder".

69

DEFICIENCY SYMPTOMS

May cause constipation, nervous disorders, edema, fatigue, lack of appetite.

FOOD SOURCES

Green Vegetables (Broccoli, Cauliflower, Lettuce, Celery), Whole Grains (Wheat, Rice, Barley), Almonds, Sunflower Seeds, Walnuts, Apples, Bananas, Lemons, Strawberries, Borage, Nettle, Yarrow, Plaintain, Comfrey Root, Walnut Leaves.

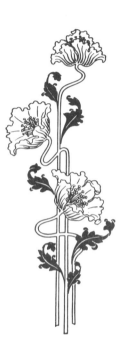

SODIUM & CHLORINE

These elements are familiar to you as common table salt. All foods have some Sodium, but unfortunately we have a tendency to cover everything with salt. This leads to many problems. Sodium and Chlorine play a part in controlling body fluids, keeping them in balance. This balance can easily become upset when we add salt to foods that already contain it. Salt attracts water and anyone on a diet would have far better results if they watched their salt intake (preferably to leave it completely alone). Prepared foods such as pickles, sauerkraut, crackers, smoked meats, all contain a great deal of Sodium Chloride. Foods that contain the least are cereals, fruits, honey, molasses, potatoes, rice.

DEFICIENCY SYMPTOMS

Hardly likely to occur considering all the foods that contain these elements; however, an imbalance of body fluids would be evident. If during the summer excess perspiration causes a slight deficiency, eating Celery, Cabbage and Watercress will replace whatever is needed.

SULPHUR

All functions performed by Sulphur have not been determined, however, we do know that it is contained in hormones which are given off by the glands of the body. It is also necessary to rebuild protein, particularly Keratin which is found in hair and skin. Sulphur is used in its synthetic form in many instances, dried fruit is treated with it. Saccharin is made with it as well as many Sulphur drugs. This synthetic form is not the same according to many nutrition experts. In fact this form has been labelled as poison to the system. Foods are the natural source and as such are valuable.

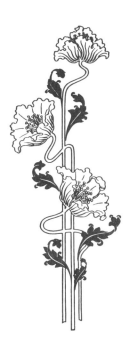

DEFICIENCY SYMPTOMS

Brittle nails, skin eruptions, hair deficiencies.

FOOD SOURCES

Meat, Fish Eggs, Cheese, Soybeans, Lentils, Kidney Beans, Cabbage, Fish, Poultry, Onions, Garlic, Swiss Chard, Watercress.

71

A WORD ABOUT FOODS

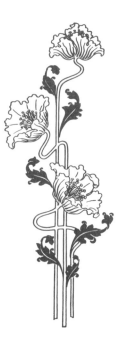

People today are becoming more aware than ever of the need to return to a more natural way of eating. Many years ago the quality of food was superior; our soil was not as contaminated with chemicals as it is today. Also the soil was allowed to rest so that it might produce healthy fruit and vegetables next time around. Whole Wheat was ground to make fresh flour and bread was baked from this providing valuable vitamins and minerals.

Rapid population growth brought with it changes. Food had to be produced faster so the new method of fertilizing with chemicals came into being. The land produced more crops but was the quality the same? White flour and refined sugar became a sign of prosperity and as people became more affluent, these items appeared on the table more often. Fruit that looked good somehow didn't taste the same. Could it be because they were picked green, then treated with chemicals to make them look ripe? How about the livestock? Even they became a target for the producers of chemicals and were shot full of drugs to promote faster growth. We are constantly reassured that chemicals in small doses do not affect us in any way, that many of the foods we buy are enriched with added vitamins. If this is so, why do people suffer from so many deficiency diseases? Why are we building more and more hospitals? We either become healthy on the foods we eat or we become listless through eating refined, devitalized, chemically treated food.

Thank goodness researchers today are taking a look at these foods and their additives and thank goodness for the return of people of all ages to the realization that live, unprocessed foods give life-giving energy to the body.

Health food stores, in the last ten years, have enjoyed new popularity as people become more aware. If you have never visited a health food store, it can be a very interesting experience. You will see products that our grandmothers used, whole grains, wholesome bread, unrefined flours, raw nuts and seeds, herbs and natural vitamins, plus an assortment of interesting books. You will probably be delighted with the helpful service and knowledgeable people who operate them. Many of them have been students of good nutrition for many years. The following products are just a few of the healthful substitutes you will find in these stores that I use in my own kitchen.

AGAR

This is a gelatin derived from sea grass. It is a rich source of minerals and contains valuable iodine. This is used in place of gelatin derived from animal sources. Available in health food stores.

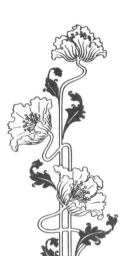

APPLE CIDER VINEGAR

Valuable to keep in the kitchen for any recipe that calls for vinegar. Excellent in salad dressings. To restore the body to a more neutral pH factor, take one tbsp. in a glass of water daily. A cupful added to the bath prevents itching and ½ cup of vinegar to ½ cup of water is a good hair rinse.

ARROWROOT FLOUR

Derived from the root of the arrowroot plant, it can be used in recipes as a substitute for baking soda, baking powder, corn starch, and wheat starch. Also good for thickening gravies.

BLACKSTRAP MOLASSES

This is the by-product of the sugar cane, rich in B vitamins, iron, and other minerals. Can be used in place of sugar. Excellent taken in hot water as a laxative.

BREWER'S YEAST

This is an excellent food that can be sprinkled on cereals or taken in a health drink (juice). Brewer's yeast contains vitamins, minerals and is a rich source of protein. It is a good source of energy and especially beneficial to vegetarians and pregnant women.

BROWN RICE FLOUR

A highly nutritious flour that contains most of the B vitamins plus minerals. If making bread, substitute 1 cup of this flour for regular flour. Gives good flavor.

BULGUR

Makes a pleasant change from rice. It is a wheat product, very tasty and much in demand in Eastern countries. Bulgur contains B vitamins, amino acids and if purchased in flour form, can be used in baking, for variety.

CAROB

Is used as a chocolate substitute. It is known as St. John's bread or honey locust. It has a delicious taste and has a high protein content. Can be purchased at health food stores in powder form or as bars or chips for baking.

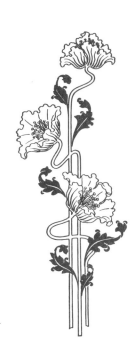

COFFEE SUBSTITUTE

There are many of these available today. Most of them are made from Barley, Chicory, Wheat or Dandelion. They do not contain caffeine and are available in instant form.

COLD PRESSED OILS

These oils are processed in a different way than most commercial oils. A cold press is used to preserve the nutrients. Also many of them do not contain preservatives. When purchasing these oils they should be refrigerated. There are many available such as Safflower, Sunflower, Sesame, Corn, Olive.

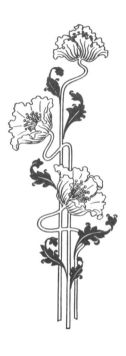

DULSE

This is a seaweed rich in iodine, minerals, vitamins. Available in powdered form, it can be used in place of salt. It is a natural product that can also be chewed in leaf form, if desired.

FRUCTOSE

Fruit sugar that looks exactly like refined white sugar, but is derived from fruits. It is extremely sweet and should be used sparingly.

GARBANZO BEANS

Sometimes called Chick-Peas. They are very high in minerals and vegetable protein and make an excellent meat substitute. A flour of these beans, called Chana, is also available which can be used in baking. A most economical survival food.

GOATS' MILK

It is said that, next to mother's milk, Goats' Milk is the best. Very easy to digest, it does not require pasteurization. Excellent for anyone with a weak digestion. Also good for some people who have allergies to Cows' Milk. Available in powder form from health food stores.

MAPLE SYRUP

Is a pure sap from the Maple tree made into a delicious syrup. It is generally used in place of sugar (like honey and molasses). More natural than the imitation syrups on the market.

MILLET SEED

An excellent source of protein, Millet can be used as a breakfast cereal. Anyone with wheat allergies usually find Millet a good substitute. Can also be used in casseroles.

MUNG BEANS

Can be sprouted and used to replace lettuce in the winter months. High in protein, vitamins and minerals. Easy to sprout and delicious to eat in sandwiches.

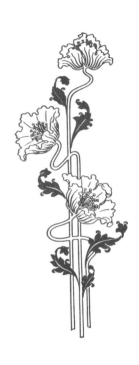

SEEDS

Sunflower, Sesame, Pumpkin, Chia, can all be ground with a nut grinder to make an excellent breakfast cereal, high in unsaturated fats, protein, vitamins and minerals. The grinder is worthwhile.

SESAME TAHINI

Ground Sesame Seeds make a paste that is high in proteins, vitamins and minerals. Can be used as a spread or to make nutritious candy. Should be used sparingly, tends to be fattening.

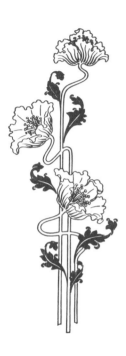

WHEAT GERM

The life of the wheat is in the germ. High in vitamins, B & E, it is also a rich source of minerals. Wheat Germ should be refrigerated and used often on cereals and in baking for extra nutrition.

WHEY POWDER

After the curds have been removed from milk, the liquid left is Whey. Very helpful to restore B vitamins. Also keeps the colon healthy, aiding digestion.

YOGURT

More digestible than milk, Yogurt is helpful to the intestinal tract. Beware of some commercial brands as sugar is added to it. It is very simple to make at home using either Cows' or Goats' milk. Especially good to replace ice cream.

BEAUTY STARTS FROM THE INSIDE OUT

Everyone likes to look attractive, male or female, young or mature. This is probably the reason that the billions of dollars spent on cosmetic items of all kinds each year, make it a top money making industry. The fact is, though, all of us can be more attractive at a fraction of the cost of commercial beauty aids. All it takes is a little experimentation in the kitchen, time and imagination. So where do we start? Since good looks actually mean a clean, healthy, vital looking skin, sparkling eyes, lively shining hair, we have to start from the inside out . . . so number one rule is one of inner cleanliness.

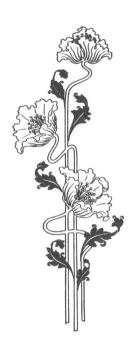

ELIMINATION

This is the number one rule of health, to keep the body working in tip top shape. If the inside is sluggish, it shows on the outside, on the skin, and through the eyes.

1. Upon arising each morning, take a glass of hot water with the juice of half a Lemon in it. This will flush the kidneys and encourage the bowel to evacuate.
2. Stretch the body, it doesn't have to be strenuous. Lie down on the floor and stretch each part of the body slowly.
3. Stand in front of an open window and breathe in slowly and deeply to the count of seven, exhale to the same count. This brings oxygen to the blood.

4. Go to the bathroom and prepare to have a bowel movement. Habit is the answer, same time each morning, eventually the body will respond and you are on your way to a good start for that sparkle in your eye.

SKIN

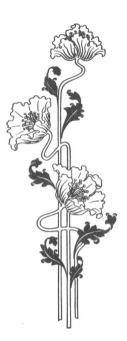

Skin should be glowing and youthful with good tone. Normal condition of the skin is moist, soft and slightly on the acid side. It is the largest organ of the body and is like the kidney, it throws off waste and protects the body. Its main functions include — protection from injury and the invasion of bacteria. It has its own built in temperature control, those little bumps that appear during exposure to extreme cold are an indication that the body is adjusting. Regulation of heat in the body is maintained by the blood and sweat glands of the skin as a protection against extreme changes of weather.

Too much time in the sun causes melanin (pigment) to come to the surface as a protective factor. Chemical substances that are rejected usually cause a flare-up on the skin, indicating all is not well. Through the nerve endings, skin responds to pressure and pain.

Absorption is a most important factor of the skin. We have to be aware of the type of cosmetics we use for it is known that hormones are taken into the body through

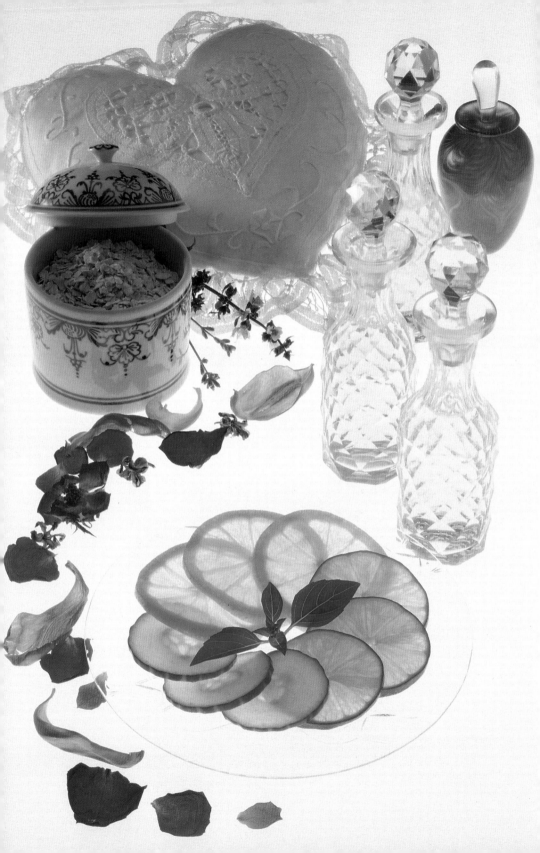

BEAUTY — THE NATURAL WAY

Apricot Oil
Almond Oil
Apple Cider Vinegar
Lime Juice
Lemons
Limes
Cucumber
Rose Petals
Oatmeal
Lavender
Basil

the skin. Certain chemicals are also absorbed so we should learn to read labels. If we don't understand them, take the time to find out what they mean. The Department of Consumer Affairs is concerned about many products allowed on the market without ingredient listing. I, personally, would never buy a cosmetic product until I had checked it out. The consumer has to be protected and everyone has a right to know what they are using. The skin is also an excretory organ which throws off waste, perspiration, carries salt and other substances out through the pores. This is, of course, the reason that dirt affects the skin. Too much sugar and salt can also cause reactions. In taking good care of your skin, there are some very basic steps needed. Routine is important.

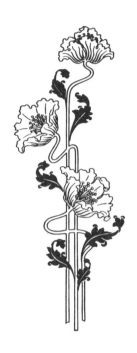

CLEANSING

Cleansing the skin is perhaps the most important, especially if you live in a city. When dirt is combined with sebum, a sluggish complexion results. Many of the commercial cleansers on the market do little to actually nourish the skin in spite of the extravagant advertising. I have done much experimenting with natural oils as cleansers and have been delighted with the results.

DRY TO NORMAL SKIN

Apply natural Apricot Oil, Peanut or Almond Oils (available at Health Stores), massage gently all over neck working up to the face always in an upward motion. Do not stretch skin underneath the eyes outward but rather work toward the nose, as the skin is especially delicate in this area. Work the Oil gently but firmly into the skin, then using a washcloth wash off with cool water several times. Notice the softness of the skin, and how effective and inexpensive the oils are with no perfumes to irritate. Other kitchen ingredients that can be used as cleansers are Mayonnaise, Buttermilk, Yogurt.

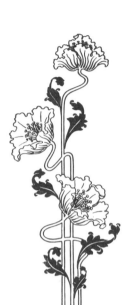

OILY SKIN

Strange as it seems, vegetable oils such as Safflower or Corn Oil can be used to clean a skin that is already oily. The big secret is in the rinsing. Five or six times with warm water should do it, then pat dry with a towel. A slice of cucumber then rubbed gently over the skin will act as an astringent and tone the skin.

STIMULATION

Since the dead cells on the skin are constantly replacing themselves, it's a good idea to help slough off the dead ones by using something coarse to buff the skin. Corn Meal is excellent, just use on a slightly dampened skin and gently massage all over the face. The skin will tingle a little but will feel very alive and fresh. Rinse thoroughly and apply moisture (either your own or a good natural commercial one). This treatment can be used on oily or dry to normal skin, once weekly to keep it in good condition.

MOISTURE

When the skin is dry, it becomes a little like parchment paper, wrinkled. Lack of moisture contributes to this condition. Also, of course, skin that has been exposed to too much sun and wind, whatever the time of year, Winter when the heat is on or Summer when the sun is out, needs an adequate moisture content to keep it young, supple and moist. Twice weekly, give yourself an avocado mask. Mash the ripe flesh, apply to skin and leave on 20 minutes (better in the bathtub, less messy). The skin responds to this treatment leaving it beautifully soft and moist. A thin film of Apricot Kernel Oil applied directly after washing keeps the skin this way.

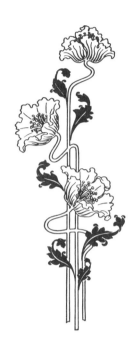

PROTECTION

Learn to protect your skin from the elements as much as possible. If you are planning a ski trip, be sure to pack some natural oils that will moisturize as well as protect your skin. Aloe Vera Gel is wonderful for this, there are some excellent creams in the health store with

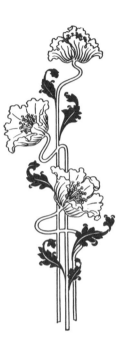

the sun screen P.A.B.A. This helps against ultra-violet rays from the sun whether on the ski run or on the beach. Be aware at all times that your skin is precious. The following recipes are effective and fun to make. Take one night a week to yourself and try whichever appeals to you. One thing is certain, you won't have wasted a great deal of money on products you don't like. Try a few of your own ideas also, you'll be surprised at some of the results.

FACIAL MASKS — DRY & NORMAL SKIN

1. 2 tbsp. cottage cheese
   1 tbsp. unpasteurized honey
   1 tbsp. yogurt
   Stir together until smooth, then apply over face and neck for 15 to 20 minutes. Rinse off thoroughly with lukewarm water several times.
2. 1 egg yolk, beaten
   ½ tsp. olive oil
   ½ tsp. lime juice
   Mix together well, leave on skin 15 minutes, wash off with water.
3. 1 egg white, beaten
   add 2 tbsp. honey
   1 tsp. lemon juice
   Leave on 20 mintues, wash off with water.

4. 2 tbsp. milk
   1 whole egg
   1 tsp. honey
   Leave on 15 minutes. Wash off with
   water.

FACIAL MASKS FOR OILY SKIN

1. 2 tbsp. oatmeal
   2 tbsp. honey
   Mix together well. Apply to skin, leave
   on 15 minutes. Wash off with warm
   water.
2. 1 egg white, beaten
   few drops lemon juice
   Mix well together. Clean skin with
   almond oil. Apply egg white mixture
   over it, leave on 10 minutes. Rinse off
   with water.
3. Mix 1 tbsp. powdered brewer's yeast to
   white of 1 egg. Beat together, leave on
   skin for 15 minutes. Rinse well.
4. Raw pulp of tomato applied to face,
   dries excessive oil.
5. Apply plain buttermilk, leave on 15
   minutes. Wash off with warm water.

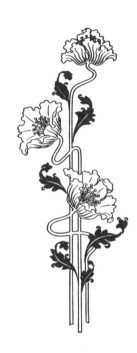

EYES

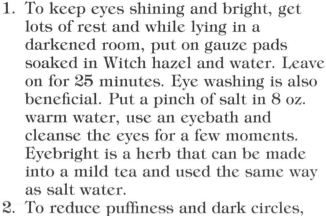

1. To keep eyes shining and bright, get lots of rest and while lying in a darkened room, put on gauze pads soaked in Witch hazel and water. Leave on for 25 minutes. Eye washing is also beneficial. Put a pinch of salt in 8 oz. warm water, use an eyebath and cleanse the eyes for a few moments. Eyebright is a herb that can be made into a mild tea and used the same way as salt water.
2. To reduce puffiness and dark circles, apply wet tea bags to the eyelid. Leave on for 15 minutes. Raw potato can also be used for this purpose.
3. For wrinkles around the eyes, use Vitamin E Oil or Apricot Kernel Oil.
4. For removing eye make-up, Olive Oil is most effective. To help eyelashes grow, smear on Castor Oil each night before retiring. To darken eyelashes, Rosemary or Sage tea brushed on does the trick.

HANDS & FEET

1. For lovely soft hands cook ½ cup oatmeal in 8 oz. water for 10 minutes. Add the juice of ½ lemon, 1 tsp. Olive Oil, rub in well.

2. Mash the pulp of a papaya, rub onto hands and gently massage in. This eliminates the dry, flaky skin. Any one of the vegetable oils make good hand lotions and, incidentally, anything good for the hands also works on the feet. Rough skin on the heels and elbows can be helped by mixing apple pulp with a little honey and applying. Rinse off and rub a little Apricot Oil in. To relax the feet, put ½ cup salt in a tub of water. Soak for 10 minutes. Feels great, walking barefoot in the grass whenever possible. It is also very relaxing. While you are watching T.V., rotate your ankles, first one way, then the other. This simple exercise keeps ankles slim and feet supple.

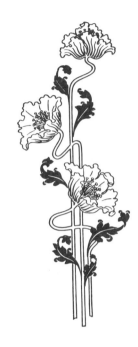

HAIR

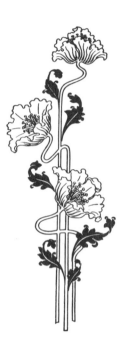

Hair is always described as a crown of glory and from a beauty point of view, hair certainly commands a great deal of time and effort. The rewards though, are instant in terms of visible results. What looks more beautiful than clean, shining, healthy hair? Here again it is a good indication of the body's state of health. Hair is composed of Keratin (protein). Diet plays a great part in the general health of the hair. Nourishment is derived from the blood supply which is dependent upon elements from the food we eat. This fact becomes very obvious when drugs are taken. The hair can become dull, lifeless and fall out by the handful. Devitalized foods such as candy, fried, greasy items, too much starch, all adversely affect the hair. A diet rich in protein, Vitamin A (vegetables, dairy products), B Complex (grains, nuts and seeds), all contribute to a beautiful head of hair. There are many other factors involved in having healthy hair. Allowing the blood to flow to the head with simple exercise is one. Absolute cleanliness with mild shampoos and avoiding harsh chemicals that do much damage to the hair and scalp is another. Use a natural bristle brush instead of the synthetic kind. The following recipes are fun to try and inexpensive to use.

OILY HAIR

Before you shampoo your hair, give it a good brush with your head bent over so that you get right underneath. Use a good herbal shampoo with Rosemary in it, if you are dark, Chamomile, if fair. After washing use a rinse of apple cider vinegar, 8 oz. to ½ pint of water, and comb thoroughly through the hair. This leaves the hair in good condition. Put a nylon stocking over the brush. Use daily on hair to absorb excessive oil.

DRY HAIR

Brush hair, then beat up 2 egg yolks, (separate whites), apply to scalp and hair. Wrap hot wet towel around the head, leave on 20 minutes. Shampoo hair twice with a good, mild pH balanced shampoo. Into the second one put 1 tsp. Wheat Germ Oil. Results . . . beautiful!

SETTING LOTION

Soak 2 tbsp. flaxseed in equal amount of water overnight. This produces a jelly-like mucilage that works so well as a setting lotion. For oily hair, skim milk can be applied with a sponge pad all over the head. Then set hair.

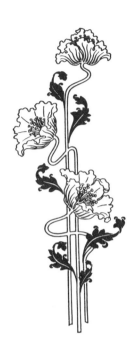

NAILS

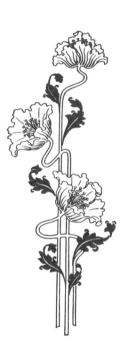

Nails are so noticeable because we use our hands constantly. Well kept nails add much to the appearance of both men and women. Whether your nails are hard or soft, a treatment 3 times weekly of warm wheat germ oil massaged into the nails, especially around the citicle, does wonders for strengthening. The nails are composed mainly of a protein substance called Keratin and, just like the skin, nails show a general indication of the state of health of an individual. Good nutrition plays a large part in the growth and state of the nails. The average growth of a nail is one eighth of an inch per month. Of more importance is the condition of the nail. Many people have complained to me that in spite of a good, balanced diet, their nails are still peeling and splitting. Assimilation seems to be the key here. In other words, is the body utilizing all of the nutrients it receives? Enzymes help to assimilate and these are found in fresh, live foods (salads and fruit). One of the best remedies I have found for nails is Comfrey. In the summertime 3 leaves a day, cut up in a salad provides both protein and calcium in a very usable form. Wintertime, Comfrey tea could be taken several times a day. Vitamin A also seems to benefit, especially when taken along with Vitamin C (both skin Vitamins), and along with Wheat Germ Oil treatment, results should be noticeable in a few weeks. Incidently, if you wear polish, apply, let it dry, then hold nails under cold water for a few minutes. Polish lasts longer.

DID YOU KNOW?

— Using a washcloth to remove creams and oils is better than using paper products? Wood fibers can irritate your skin. Notice when you have a cold how sore your nose gets? Be sure to have a good supply though, of clean washcloths.

— That using excessively hot water tends to dry the skin out and adds to aging? Lukewarm is better.

— By applying cream while the skin is still a little damp after washing, the moisture is absorbed by the skin easier and is more effective.

— Castor Oil is great for eyelashes, encourages growth.

— Deodorant sometimes irritates because of allergic reaction to the chemical ingredients used. Chapparral tea (used externally) or dusting with plain baking soda will give protection without the side effects.

— For large pores on the nose, whip up an eggwhite, add a few drops of lemon juice, apply with a paintbrush. Leave on 20 minutes (3 times weekly).

— Chapped lips can be avoided by applying Vaseline, Apricot Oil or Honey before applying lipstick (if worn).

— Liver spots will fade if you faithfully use fresh onion juice (apply directly) or buttermilk. These are natural bleaching agents.

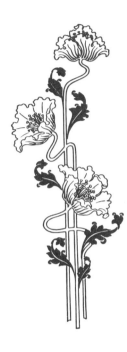

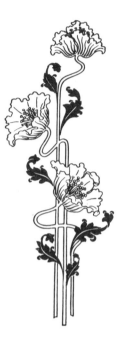

— It is wise to test all cosmetic items (including those you make) on an area inside the forearm (behind the elbow). If you have a rash in 20 minutes, do not use. This takes a little time but is well worth the effort.

— You can make a natural mouthwash by putting 1 tsp. of sassafras with 8 oz. water, boil together, let cool, then use to rinse mouth.

— Cocoa Butter rubbed on the tummy, while pregnant, helps to prevent stretch marks.

— By using a loofah sponge in the shower each day and working in a circular upward motion, your circulation will improve, skin impurities fade away and you feel more energetic.

— By taking a bath to which has been added 1 lb. sea salt, 1 lb. baking soda, all those aches and pains disappear.

— Instead of using costly bath oil, any vegetable oil such as Safflower, Sunflower, Peanut, will do the same thing. Also, if you put your favorite herbs in a little cheesecloth and hold under running water (Rose petals, Lavender, Basil), the water smells delightful.

INDEX

INDULGE A FRIEND

Order **Basic Herbs and Simple Remedies** or **The Herb Patch** at $11.95 per book plus $1.50 for shipping and handling for each copy.

The Herb Patch _____ x $11.95 = _____

Basic Herbs and Simple Remedies _____ x $11.95 = _____

Postage and Handling Charge _____ x $ 1.50 = _____

In Canada, add 7% G.S.T. _____(subtotal x .07)= _____

Total enclosed _____ = _____

U.S. and international orders payable in U.S. funds / Price is subject to change

NAME _____

STREET _____

CITY _____ PROV./STATE _____

COUNTRY _____ POSTAL CODE/ZIP _____

Please make cheque or money order payable to:

NuYu Enterprises
Box 8432, Station F
Calgary, Alberta
T2J 2V5

U.S. Orders:
NuYu Enterprises
P.O. Box 16200 - 313
Mesa, Arizona
85201

For fund-raising or volume purchases, contact NUYU ENTERPRISES.
Please allow 3-4 weeks for delivery.

INDULGE A FRIEND

Order **Basic Herbs and Simple Remedies** or **The Herb Patch** at $11.95 per book plus $1.50 for shipping and handling for each copy.

The Herb Patch _____ x $11.95 = _____

Basic Herbs and Simple Remedies _____ x $11.95 = _____

Postage and Handling Charge _____ x $ 1.50 = _____

In Canada, add 7% G.S.T. _____(subtotal x .07)= _____

Total enclosed _____ = _____

U.S. and international orders payable in U.S. funds / Price is subject to change

NAME _____

STREET _____

CITY _____ PROV./STATE _____

COUNTRY _____ POSTAL CODE/ZIP _____

Please make cheque or money order payable to:

NuYu Enterprises
Box 8432, Station F
Calgary, Alberta
T2J 2V5

U.S. Orders:
NuYu Enterprises
P.O. Box 16200 - 313
Mesa, Arizona
85201

For fund-raising or volume purchases, contact NUYU ENTERPRISES.
Please allow 3-4 weeks for delivery.